Rhythm Sticks Cardio for Seniors

Realize Your Fitness With Fun and Rhythm

Faith Watson

losses, direct or indirect, that are incurred as a result of the use of the information contained within this document, including, but not limited to, errors, omissions, or inaccuracies.

Table of Contents

Introduction

If you're anything like me, you get bored with regular workouts. You recognize that working out is important for both your physical and mental health, but the idea of going to the gym and walking on the treadmill sounds teeth-grindingly boring to you. So, you need something a lot more fun, something that can keep you engaged but also provide you with a proper workout. Enter rhythm sticks cardio, the kind of workout that's as entertaining as it is beneficial, at least for me. Rhythm sticks can provide you with a rather unexpected kind of workout. It's certainly not one that you hear people talk about a lot. In this regard, it's a bit like aerial arts or ribbons, both of which are incredibly aesthetic methods of exercising. This is another similarity that the two have with rhythm sticks cardio, a fact you might have noticed yourself if you're acquainted with this sport. If you're not, you might be wondering what rhythm sticks even are.

Rhythm sticks are essentially a pair of notched or plain wooden sticks that you strike together to produce percussive sounds. As you might have guessed from the name, they're great for helping you to improve and maintain your sense of rhythm. This is part of the reason they are an ideal cardio option for seniors. Rhythm isn't just important for your ability to dance, after all. Having a good sense of rhythm can help you understand the events that are going on around you in real time by being able to keep up with them. It can also help you maintain your hand–eye coordination and manage dialogues and conversations well. It can even keep you from missing a step as you're walking down the street or changing up your pace, and thus prevent you injuring yourself. From running to drinking a cup of tea, your sense of rhythm plays a part in everything that you do, which is why you want to keep it in tip-top shape (Baarøy, 2020).

Rhythm sticks cardio can help you with other things besides your sense of rhythm too. For instance, it can increase your spatial awareness, which will go a long way toward reducing your risk of falls and tumbles. For seniors, something as simple as a fall can have grievous consequences. Every year, approximately 36 million seniors end up having to go to the ER or to see their physicians because of injuries sustained during a fall; 32,000 of those cases sadly result in the patient's death. Meanwhile, one out of every five falls results in either a head injury or a broken bone, and more than 95% of all hip fractures are caused by falling (Baarøy, 2020). Falls partly happen because as you grow older your propensity to misjudge the space between things increases. Simultaneously, you become prone to tripping over things because you didn't see them there. This all has to do with your decreasing sense of spatial awareness. This does not have to be the case, though. You can improve your spatial awareness, just as you can improve any sense or muscle, through rhythm sticks cardio.

Speaking of muscles, since rhythm sticks cardio is a workout, it can prevent the muscle mass loss that comes with aging. Once you hit your 30s, you start losing something between three and eight percent of your muscle mass every 10 years. When you get to be over 60, you start losing even more than that (Volpi et al., 2004). This is actually another reason seniors fall down a lot. Loss of muscle mass means weaker muscles, and weaker muscles mean having a harder time keeping upright, especially when you lose your balance. Loss of muscle mass also means loss of motor skills, at least to a degree. It's a good thing, then, that rhythm sticks cardio is known to improve your motor skills, including your ability to grasp things, change up your direction and pace really quickly, and more.

Assuming you're taking part in group sessions, rhythm sticks cardio can help you get better at teamwork. You will need to have your own sticks in your hands for this and then pair up with someone. This makes rhythm sticks cardio both a really fun activity to do with a partner or a friend, and a wonderful environment to meet new people and forge friendships with them (Leslie, 2014).

For a sport that's relatively new, rhythm sticks cardio sure seems to have a lot of different iterations. There are the typical, though no less fun, examples like dance choreographies. Then there are the rather unexpected and innovative ones, like cardio drumming, which has become a growing trend across the country over the years. Done with a sturdy base, like a large bucket, and Pilates balls, which serve as the "drums," this version of the exercise provides people with a real opportunity to rock out and seems to pair especially well with *We Will Rock You*. Whatever version you go with, though, you end up burning a lot of calories. How can you not with all that banging about? This is true even for a more stationary version of the sport, like cardio drumming, since it involves standing straight-backed while bending slightly over your drum, which keeps your abs engaged.

Generally speaking, rhythm sticks cardio provides you with a full-body workout. So, it's not just about striking your sticks against one another. There are lunges and squats incorporated into your routine, as well as choreographed steps. The workouts sometimes get so intense that your heart rate can jump to 190 beats per minute, once you've become a pro. Before you ask, that's a good thing. Cardio exercises, by their definition, get your heart rate elevated. You want this to be the case because it strengthens your heart. Your heart is a muscle and, like any muscle, it only gets stronger the more of a workout it gets. When you do cardio—or aerobics as it's otherwise known—you increase your heart rate, meaning the rate at which your heart is beating, at least initially. Over time, your heart becomes able to pump more oxygen to your body with less effort. This means your resting heart rate—the rate at which your heart beats while you're resting—goes down, allowing your heart to transport more oxygen and nutrients to the cells throughout your body with much less effort.

This is just the tip of the tip of the iceberg, really. Cardio has many other advantages to offer seniors, including (Fetters, 2018):

- lower blood pressure

- lower cholesterol levels

- lower risk of developing heart disease

- weight loss

- increased lung capacity

- lower blood sugar levels

- stronger bones

- lowered stress and anxiety levels

- a stronger immune system

Seeing as rhythm sticks cardio is an aerobic activity, all these benefits apply to it as well. Coupled with the benefits that are unique to it, it's clear to see how broad and useful a fitness workout rhythm sticks makes for, especially for seniors. What are the different ways you can incorporate rhythm sticks into your workout sessions, though? How can you make it so that you reap all the advantages this sport has to offer? While you're at it, how can you go about ensuring your workout sessions are as safe as possible? Speaking as someone who has been into rhythm sticks cardio for many years, the answers to these questions are things I'm intimately familiar with. Hence, *Rhythm Sticks Cardio for Seniors* will cover all this and more. It will introduce you to a sport that is easy to pick up, fun to do, and incredibly helpful to you in a variety of ways. It will show you how you can ease into this workout, as well as become an expert at it, all while making new friends and enjoying your time. All you have to do for this is to read on.

Chapter 1:

Understanding Seniors'

Fitness Needs

Before we can delve into how rhythm sticks cardio can be done and why it's one of the best sports seniors can pick up, we must first understand why seniors need to work out in the first place. There's a widespread belief, you see, that people over a certain age shouldn't work out because there is a high chance they'll end up hurting themselves. Seniors' propensity for falling and thus injuring themselves is likely to blame for this. This belief, however, couldn't be less true. Seniors absolutely do need to work out, and they need to do so around 5 days a week, every week. In fact, they need this more than younger people do. It is this level of activity, not lack thereof, that will keep them from injuring themselves. It's also this level of activity that will keep their immune system, heart, lungs, and other organs strong and in tip-top shape. According to the Centers for Disease Control and Prevention (CDC), working out regularly can delay any age-related health problems seniors might experience. It can make their muscles stronger, thereby ensuring they become less accident prone and more independent in their everyday lives.

The CDC specifically recommends that adults over the age of 65 (CDC, 2021):

- engage in moderate-intensity workouts for 150 minutes per week, which equals just 30 minutes every day for 5 days out of the week, or

- engage in high-intensity workouts for 75 minutes per week, which would equal 15 minutes of activity per day for 5 days out of the week

For the record, moderate-level cardio workouts are made up of exercises that raise your heart rate and breathing rates and make you feel warmer. At a moderate level of intensity, you should still be able to talk to someone next to you while working out but you shouldn't be able to, say, sing. Activities such as brisk walking, biking, hiking, and dancing would all count as moderate-level exercise. So would rhythm sticks cardio, though you can kick up its intensity level to high if you want to. Exercises that count as high intensity are those that get you breathing hard and fast. They're the kinds of activities that have your heart positively drumming and, if you're engaged in this kind of workout, then you shouldn't be able to say more than a couple of words without having to catch your breath (National Health Service, 2021). Typically, activities like running, swimming, and walking up the stairs count as high-intensity exercises.

So, why exactly do seniors need to work out regularly? The answer to this question lies in the physical and even mental changes that happen within the human body as it ages. It also has to do with the impact that regular workouts can have on those very changes.

Age-Related Changes in the Body

Aging is something we all have to deal with eventually. There's no changing or going around that. However, how fast we age and how much aging affects our bodies is entirely up to us. There are several things you can do to slow down the effects of aging and make sure that your body remains strong and healthy as you get older. Regular exercise is chief among these. Take your immune system, for example. As you age, your immune system gets weaker because your bone marrow starts producing fewer immune cells such as your T and B cells. When you exercise regularly, however, you slow down this process—so much so that studies have shown that the immune systems of seniors who regularly exercise end up being as strong as those of people who are in their 20s (Montecino-Rodriguez et al., 2013).

That's not all, since regular exercise has also been found to slow down your biological clock. We all have DNA, as you know, and that DNA is found in tiny little things called chromosomes. Chromosomes have these things called telomeres at their ends. Think of telomeres as tiny little caps. Now, as your cells multiply, so do your chromosomes. Each time a chromosome splits to make a new one, those telomeres become shorter. Thus, the more you age, the shorter your telomeres become. By the time you get to the end of your life, you get close to running out of telomeres too. This means that there is a kind of parallel, corresponding relationship between your telomeres and your life span, which is why you want your telomeres to be as long as humanly possible. The longer they are, the longer you will live (Tucker, 2017).

The best way to make sure you have long telomeres that will last you a long, long time is to exercise regularly. That's right, regular exercise prevents you from losing too many of your telomeres over the years, to the point that it adds, at minimum, an additional 9 years to your life.

Of course, you don't want just to live longer but to live well. Exercising regularly ensures you are able to do this too. This is partly because it improves your overall mood, your ability to focus and pay attention to things, and your memory. Exercise slows down the rate at which your brain ages, which is when you see an improvement in all these different areas. The brain of someone who works out several times a week ages 10 times more slowly than someone who leads a more sedentary lifestyle (Suzuki, 2017).

Meanwhile, exercise helps aging seniors to build muscle. This is important because people lose a lot of muscle mass as they age. This is a condition known as sarcopenia, and workouts are the best way to prevent it. When you work out, you build more muscle, so even if you lose some to aging, you have more than enough remaining to pull open a heavy door or climb a set of stairs. This is why exercise increases your mobility and independence in old age. The fact that exercising increases your bone density plays a part in this too.

When you're young, your body breaks down your old bones and replaces them regularly with new bone tissue. When you hit age 30, though, it stops generating new bone mass to make up for the loss. You start feeling the effects of this in your 40s and 50s, since by then you'll be losing more bone mass than you can create. If this goes on for long enough, you can develop osteoporosis, otherwise known as brittle bone disease, a condition that makes it all too easy for you to fracture and break your bones. Osteoporosis is partly to blame for all those fractures seniors end up with after experiencing a fall. That being said, this is only true for seniors who don't exercise. Those who do get to keep generating more bone mass, even well into their 70s and 80s. Thus, they get to make sure their bones remain strong and sturdy and don't suffer the same health consequences their sedentary counterparts do (Seegert, 2021).

Exercise can be very helpful to you if you already have a condition like osteoporosis or arthritis too. People who have such conditions usually don't want to move about, and understandably so. They operate under the assumption that moving around will worsen the pain and discomfort that they are in. Exercise, however, will do the very opposite of this. Regular exercise—or, at least, arthritis-friendly exercise (which, for the record, rhythm sticks cardio is)—helps alleviate this kind of joint and bone pain. It prevents the joints from becoming stiff and keeps them well lubricated and therefore able to move around freely. This in turn makes movement itself easier, while reducing pain.

Joint problems and bone conditions are just one example among the many diseases that exercise can prevent. There's also heart conditions, and that makes sense when you think about it. When you exercise, you give your heart a good workout. Since your heart is a muscle, this exercise proves good for it and strengthens your heart and your cardiovascular system in the long run. In keeping with this, your likelihood of developing other diseases related to your cardiovascular system—like hypertension, diabetes, and obesity—goes down as well. On top of that, exercise lowers your chances of developing various types of cancer, including colon cancer of all things, and other, similar chronic diseases.

A final benefit of exercise is that it alleviates any stress and anxiety you might be feeling and keeps it from becoming chronic. It floods your system with endorphins and serotonin, which make you feel good instead. This elevates both your day-to-day mood and your overall mood. These effects last well into your 60s and 70s, thus preventing disorders such as depression and generalized anxiety disorder, ensuring you have good mental health in the years to come (*Working It Out*, 2019).

Exercise Safety Considerations for Seniors

To be honest, a whole separate book could be written about the myriad of benefits that regular exercise has to offer seniors. The main draw from all this is that seniors not only *can* work out regularly, but *should*, so long as they take certain safety measures and precautions, of course. The thing is, a 60-year-old individual's body is not the same as a 20-year-old's. So, while a 60-year-old man or woman can work out, they cannot push their bodies to the limit the way they could when they were 20. Their body simply will not allow it, at least not without sustaining an injury of some sort. Now, it's true that you want to work up some sweat while you're working out. You don't want to overdo it, though. You want your workout to be challenging but not overwhelming. Otherwise, you risk overworking your muscles and tasking them with more than they can handle. This can easily result in you pulling a muscle or even fracturing a bone.

Your first safety consideration when working out, then, is to pay close attention to what your body is telling you, and to meet its needs accordingly. If your body is telling you that the exercises you're doing are too hard at the moment by using muscle tremors and pain as signals, then you must immediately stop. You must also reduce the intensity of your exercises. One thing you can do to ensure that this never happens is to start slow and small and then build up the intensity. With cardio exercises like rhythm sticks, that can mean keeping the tempo relatively low and then increasing its speed as time goes on. This way, you can gradually get your muscles used to all that movement, instead of going from 0 to 100 in the blink of an eye, which will only increase your odds of injuring yourself.

The best way to go about doing this is to start your workouts with a warm-up and stretching period. For the record, stretching does not count as warming up. In fact, doing stretches without properly warming up first can cause you to strain something. What you should do instead is do some proper warm-up moves, which we will cover in chapters to come. This way, you can slowly raise your body temperature and increase the amount of blood that's being pumped to your muscles. Since more blood means more oxygen, you'll ensure your muscles get all the oxygen they need to perform well during your workout. As an added bonus, by warming up you can strengthen the connection between your muscles and your nerves, which will help you to execute whatever movements you have to make more efficiently.

Another way to make sure you don't push yourself too much is to take regular breaks throughout your workout. Breaks are very important when exercising, no matter what age you are. Failing to stop and take a short rest while exercising actually increases your risk of experiencing a heart attack by overworking your heart, as well as having a stroke or going through some other, similar cardiovascular issue (May, 2019). On top of that, breaks give you ample opportunity to drink water and thus hydrate yourself, the importance of which cannot be overstated. You can end up experiencing a lot of very unpleasant symptoms and side effects when you don't keep yourself hydrated while you work out, such as headaches, muscle cramps, and bodily weakness. You can also find that you've gotten dizzy, which can cause you to take a tumble and injure yourself, thanks to your suddenly dropping blood pressure. You should be sure to drink plenty of water, then, whenever you take a break during your workouts. One thing you shouldn't do during your breaks, though, is to sit down and remain still. Instead, you should be engaging in some moderate level of activity like walking around. By doing that, you can lower your heart and breathing rates slowly and make it easier for your body to recover.

Meanwhile, you should have rest periods between your workout sessions too. These periods, known as recovery time, are important because they give your muscles the time they need to repair their tissues, and your body the time it needs to restore your normal hormone levels and replenish your energy stores. If you're over 50 years old, then ideally you want to have a 48-hour recovery period between your cardio workout sessions. You can engage in other kinds of workouts—like strength or balance exercises, which are things you should be doing anyway—during those days (Prvulovic, 2023).

Not wearing appropriate gear for your workout and not being mindful of your surroundings are among the chief reasons seniors get injured while working out. As a rule, you don't want to wear any type of loose clothing that can get caught on the things around you. You want to wear well-fitting, comfortable clothes that are easy to move around in. While you're at it, you want to make sure that the materials your clothes are made of don't cause you to become overheated. You also don't want to wear shoes that don't fit you well. If they pinch your feet or if they're a bit too big, they're not the right shoes for you. Wearing them can increase your chances of tripping, falling, breaking a bone, or even suffering a head injury and a concussion. Speaking of tripping, you need to be aware of what's around you at all times while you're working out. You don't want your grandchild's toys to be strewn about the place while you're working out or for there to be stray items here and there that can cause you to slip. You should always check your environment carefully before beginning any workout session to eliminate such possibilities.

You already know that warming up is an important part of working out safely, but did you know that cooling down is as well? Just as warming up gets you to warm up your body and muscles gradually, cooling down gets you to do the reverse slowly as well. By doing cool-down exercises, you gradually return your heart and breathing rate to what they were before your session began. In doing so, you give yourself more time to adjust and reduce your likelihood of somehow injuring yourself (Mayo Clinic Staff, 2021).

There are two other things you can do to ensure your workout sessions remain as safe as possible. The first is to get enough sleep every night. Seniors need between 7 and 9 hours of sleep every night. On days that you work out, however, you might need as many as 10 hours of sleep. It's important that you meet this requirement. This is what your body needs to properly regain its strength and energy. It's all that strength and energy that you will use in your workout sessions. Without enough sleep, not only do you effectively become weaker, but your ability to concentrate on what you're doing goes down as well. As a result, you become more prone to making mistakes while working out and having an accident that would result in an injury.

The second thing you need to do is to use any and all assisted devices you need while you are working out.

There's nothing embarrassing about having to get some support from the back of a nearby, sturdy chair, or your walker for that matter. Far from being unnecessary, such measures are vital for ensuring your strength and well-being. They can keep you from falling and make it easier for you to maintain the right posture when exercising. Since maintaining the wrong posture is another prime way you can injure yourself, assisted devices can be considered a major preventative measure. They can also be considered a part of tailoring fitness programs to suit your needs.

Tailoring Fitness Programs for Senior Participants

Exercise and fitness programs for seniors need to account for their needs. As such, they need to be tailored for them, at an individual level. Fitness programs that are tailored for seniors must seek to promote healthy aging. Healthy aging promotes wellness and health as people age. It ensures that they remain active and able to function as independently as possible. Fitness programs for seniors need to aim for this, as opposed to unrealistic goals like stopping aging altogether.

A senior citizen who has high functionality is someone whose body is still able to perform various tasks (Fahmy, n.d.). To be fair, everyone's range is different in this regard. Something that might be easy to do for one person might be a lot harder for another, and that's alright. This is why fitness programs need to first gauge an individual's fitness level and take that as a baseline, in order to tailor the program to the person they are dealing with. Only by doing this can they determine what level that individual should start at and what their personal fitness goals should be, which is why such programs need to run fitness tests on their participants.

Fitness tests or assessments for seniors typically have them perform basic moves like sitting down on and standing up from a chair, balancing on one leg for a period of time, or performing a squat. Such movements allow the test-giver to assess the test-taker's range of movement, balance, and overall strength. This information is then used to adapt any movements used in the fitness program in which they'll be participating. For example, if a senior is taking a rhythm sticks cardio class and the instructor realizes that they aren't able to perform squats well, but squats are a part of the routine they've devised, then that instructor can modify things a bit and have the participant perform a half-squat instead.

Tailoring fitness programs for seniors can require a bit of creativity and ingenuity on the instructor's part. After all, the goal will be to provide participants with moves that are neither too challenging nor too easy for them to do. At the same time, tailored fitness programs should prioritize posture, gait, and balance, which are vital for healthy aging. A 30-minute class should consist roughly of a warm-up and stretching session, cardio movements that get the blood circulation going, strength-training moves, balance exercises, and a cool-down and stretching session (*Fitness for Seniors*, 2013). Luckily, rhythm sticks cardio inherently features all these things.

Why Rhythm Sticks Are Ideal for Seniors' Cardio Workouts

There are a number of different fitness programs that have been tailored specifically for seniors. Of these, rhythm sticks cardio is the most ideal form of workout that a senior citizen can go for. There are many different reasons for this. For starters, rhythm sticks cardio is as easy to do as it is physically demanding. Coupled with typically upbeat music, it includes a lot of movement and ensures that participants exercise different muscle groups at all times. Regular fitness moves like squats, dance steps and movements, and striking the sticks that the person next to you is holding are all examples of things you could do during a cardio session.

The broad range of rhythm sticks cardio movements can be done at varying levels of intensity. This allows for participants to switch things up as they practice, going from high to low or lower intensity as needed (Loncaric, 2022). It also keeps things more entertaining and engaging for participants. That the movements are low impact, for the most part, makes it possible for those taking part to keep going without putting any strain on their body or joints. Despite this, it certainly gets your heart rate elevated, especially when you're drumming, and provides you with a full-body workout.

That rhythm sticks cardio is such a versatile form of exercise means it has a great many benefits to offer you. One benefit is that it helps you to burn a lot of calories, which is why it's considered a very effective way to both manage your weight and lose some if you want to. Another is that it raises your overall level of endurance. This is because rhythm sticks cardio is a continuous form of exercise. This means that, barring any water breaks you take in between, it's the kind of workout where one movement flows into another, keeping you active for the entirety of the session. This is great for your heart, as it strengthens it even more and thus ensures your cardiovascular health (Barr, 2023).

One of the best, non-health-related benefits of rhythm sticks cardio is how inclusive it is. Everyone can participate in the sport, regardless of whether they are 7 years old, 17, or even 70. People from all fitness levels can participate in the sport too, since it can easily be tailored to their level and needs. Rhythm sticks cardio is also very accommodating for people with restricted mobility, which makes it a good workout to try if you are in a wheelchair, for example. This is partly why there is a seated version of the exercises. There are also versions that have you use softer sticks for lower impact or softer music to accommodate your fitness level, or that allow you to take breaks frequently, if that's what you need. With all these benefits at hand, it's no wonder that rhythm sticks cardio has become a growing trend, which means that you are in good company.

To really be part of that company, though, you're going to have to get some proper equipment. Mainly, you're going to have to choose the perfect rhythm sticks for you.

Chapter 2:

Getting Started—Choosing

Your Rhythm Sticks

The primary equipment that you are going to need for rhythm sticks cardio is… rhythm sticks! Who would have thought? This might seem like a simple matter, but that's not the case to the extent you might think. There are a lot of factors you have to consider when you're choosing your rhythm sticks, you see. Before we delve into those factors, let's first define what rhythm sticks are. Rhythm sticks are wooden sticks that resemble claves, which are a kind of percussion instrument that are 7–9 inches long and about 0.9 inches in diameter. They can be a little bigger or shorter than that, though. It's not uncommon to find rhythm sticks that are 1.8 inches in diameter, for instance, which is double the usual size. All come in pairs and obviously the sticks that make up each pair are the same size. Rhythm sticks can be either ribbed or smooth. They can be made of wood or plastic and you can go with either, depending on the kind of sound you want to achieve.

Types and Sizes of Rhythm Sticks

Since there are a number of rhythm sticks to choose from, let's start with the progenitor of them all: the **Lummi stick**. Rhythm sticks are actually a derivative of a Native American percussive instrument called the Lummi stick. These were created by the Lummi native people, who are based in the Pacific Northwest, near Washington. They are 0.75 inches in diameter and about 7 inches long.

Then there are **traditional rhythm sticks**, the kind that are most often used in schools these days. These sticks tend to be around 12 inches long, though they are about as thick as Lummi sticks. Often, they're painted blue, though they can be any color. They are either fluted or cylindrical.

Claves technically count as rhythm sticks and can certainly be used in rhythm sticks cardio. Claves are a kind of percussive instrument that are about an inch thick in diameter and 8–10 inches long. Usually, they're made of wood or plastic, but lately fiberglass and plastic ones have been hitting the market too. They make a rather distinct clicking noise when you strike them against one another. Sometimes they can be hollow in the middle, which can make them sound even better.

You can actually use **regular sticks you find outside** for rhythm sticks cardio too. The one rule to follow here is that the ones you choose should be roughly the same size. You'll notice that they make a much quieter sound when you strike them against one another. You may also end up with splinters when you're using such sticks, especially if they snap, which is a very real possibility. They do have quite a natural and cool texture, though, which could add a whole new level to your practice.

You can also use **pool noodles**, which are those giant rolls you'd typically use in a swimming pool. You wouldn't use the whole thing, of course. Instead, you'd cut off baton-sized chunks and use those. Obviously, these will be much wider in diameter. They're a great option for individuals who have weaker grips and are therefore prone to dropping things. They also look really colorful and aesthetic and are much less likely to hurt someone nearby should you happen to strike them accidentally.

Alternatively, you can **make your very own rhythm sticks**. To do this, you are going to need (Hanna, 2022):

- a ¾-inch PVC pipe

- colorful permanent markers

- a roll of paper towels

- a PVC pipe cutter

- medium-grit sandpaper

To start, you need to cut your PVC pipe into 12-inch-long pieces using your PVC pipe cutter. As you do, make sure that their ends aren't jagged and that your sticks are dry and clean. If you notice that the ends are jagged, you can take out your sandpaper and use it to lightly sand them down. That done, you can move onto decorating your sticks, and this is where the permanent markers come in.

Factors to Consider When Choosing Rhythm Sticks

So, how do you choose what kind of rhythm stick you want to go with? You start by considering how thick you want the stick you're holding to be. As a rule, your sticks should feel comfortable in your hands. If the ones you are holding feel too thick and too long, then odds are they're not the right ones for you—and that's perfectly alright. The thickness of the rhythm sticks you're using and how comfortable they feel in your hands will play a direct role in whether you're able to grip them correctly. So, it's important that you make the right choice for you, rather than go with the pair that you think you are supposed to choose.

The same rule applies to the length of your rhythm sticks, which is another factor to consider. How long or short do you want your sticks to be? If you are going to be striking your sticks against your partners', for example, opting for sticks that are on the longer side is probably a good idea. That way you can avoid accidentally striking your partners' fingers. Using longer sticks may also reduce the impact the strikes you make will have on your wrists, at least to some degree. Hence, this is another factor to bear in mind.

Still another is what kind of texture you want. Rhythm sticks are usually made from wood, fiberglass, or plastic.

The kind of material they're made from affects how they sound when you strike them against one another and against other things. It also impacts how they feel in your hands. If you want to find the ones that work best for you, then you have to try a couple of different models, including ones that are fully smooth and ones that are grooved. Test out sticks made from different materials to see whether you like their texture. Hit them against one another and try to determine whether this sound would be pleasing to you. You are going to have to hear them a lot in your cardio sessions, after all. Speaking of sound, you need to give some thought to whether you want your rhythm sticks to be hollow or not. This factor will impact how your sticks sound as well.

A final factor to take a look at when choosing your rhythm sticks is color. Rhythm sticks cardio can be a rather aesthetic sport. So, it stands to reason that you'd want aesthetically pleasing equipment for it. It's a good thing, then, that rhythm sticks can come in a variety of colors. You can go with a light blue (which is the typical color Lummi sticks adopt), red, orange, green, or any other color you'd like. If you'd rather keep things simple, you can opt for plain wood-colored ones as well. Whatever your choice, it's important that you go with the sticks that feel, sound, and look the best to you.

Ensuring Comfort and Safety During Workouts

There are a couple of rules you need to keep in mind to ensure your safety when doing rhythm sticks cardio. Some of these may be obvious to you; others may be news. Regardless of which is which, to ensure your comfort and safety during your workouts you have to:

- always be mindful of your posture and grip so that you can execute movements correctly and without injuring yourself

- be careful where you tap your sticks against one another so that you don't catch your fingers

- always grip your sticks from the bottom ends to reduce your risk of hitting your fingers when you strike them together

- remember to take breaks regularly throughout your practice so that you don't overtax yourself

- drink plenty of water during your breaks

- go with a tempo that suits your current fitness level

- adjust any movements to your specific needs and limits and use assisted devices as necessary

So long as you follow these guidelines and the instructions your instructor gives you, you should be perfectly safe and you'll end up greatly enjoying yourself.

Chapter 3:

Warming Up With Rhythm

Sticks

A workout session—any workout session—begins with a good warm-up. This is just as true for rhythm sticks cardio as it is for any other sport, assuming you want to reduce your chances of sustaining an injury of some sort. A good cardio session is one that lasts between 10 and 15 minutes and gradually increases your heart rate and body temperature. It involves various dynamic movements that get you to actively move your joints. This prepares them for everything that they'll be doing during your actual workout session. Now, you might be tempted to skip your warm-up sessions or cut them short and, thus, get straight to the good part. It's vital that you do not do this, though. You might be skeptical as to how effective warming up really is. After all, what's the big deal? So, before we cover the various warm-up exercises you can do with rhythm sticks, let's first establish why warm-ups are so important in the first place.

The Importance of a Proper Warm-Up

When you exercise, you end up actively using your muscles and providing them with a challenge. This is a given. If you dive into an exercise session without warming up first, you'll basically end up catching your muscles by surprise. As a result, your body will remain unprepared for the physiological changes that will accompany your training. Your muscles will struggle to get more oxygen so that they can do all that's expected of them. So, your heart will kick up from 0 to 100—or try to, anyway. This puts a real strain on it and leaves you breathless. It may even result in you experiencing some pain in your chest. The real danger with not warming up, though, is that, deprived as they will be of the extra oxygen they need to perform their job, your muscles will become unable to handle the strain that's placed on them (Cordier, 2018). Since they're rendered weaker and more inflexible, it will become all too easy for you to pull a muscle or sustain another kind of similar injury.

Warm-ups raise your body temperature gradually and supply your muscles with more oxygen in the process. This makes them stronger and more flexible. Actually, warm-ups make your whole body, including your joints, more flexible as well. This is especially true when you stretch a little after your warm-up exercises. Flexibility further reduces your chances of injuring yourself as you work out. It ensures that you won't strain yourself if you overstretch when you're performing a particular move or something like that.

A final benefit of warming up is that it mentally prepares you for the workout you're going to be starting. Being mentally prepared for your fitness session is important because it can stop you from quitting halfway. It's something that can push you to perform your best and push past your limits, even and especially when the going gets tough. In the process, it can make you get more into your workout and enjoy it a great deal more.

Dynamic Warm-Up Exercises With Rhythm Sticks

Good warm-up exercises are ones that get you moving about and that raise your body temperature gradually. Given that, you have to start slowly and then up the intensity of your exercise moves. A typical warm-up session for rhythm sticks cardio lasts about 10 minutes. It starts with smaller and slower movements and makes them bigger and faster over time. A typical warm-up session might start by having you walk about or march in place with your sticks in your hands. Then, you might have to perform a variety of movements with your sticks to warm your entire body up. Some of the most typical warm-up exercises you'll have to perform are (Hanna, 2022):

- **taps**, where you lean down to strike your stick or sticks against the ground in front of you

- **L taps,** where you lean to the left with your feet shoulder-width apart to tap the ground with a stick on your left side

- **R taps**, where you lean to the right with your feet shoulder-width apart to tap the ground with a stick on your right side

- **ends**, where you strike the bottom ends of your sticks, which are known as their ends, against the ground in front of you

- **clicks**, where you strike the tips of the sticks against one another in front of you

- **overhead clicks**, where you strike your sticks together above your head

- **claps**, where you hit the lengths of your sticks before you

- **cross taps**, where you cross your arms in front of you and then tap the ground with the sticks you are still holding

- **flips**, where you carefully throw your sticks into the air and catch them

- **throws**, where you throw a stick to your partner to catch and your partner throws theirs to you

A routine warm-up session might have you start marching or jogging in place, then performing a tap, a clap, an L tap, a clap, an R tap, a clap, and a cross tap, for instance, then have you repeat that pattern twice. It can use any other combination of these movements too, with different patterns. Most likely, those patterns will pick up more and more speed as you go along, until you've worked up a little bit of a sweat and warmed up your body sufficiently.

If you're doing cardio drumming specifically, your warm-up may have you focus on simple drumming patterns so that you can engage and warm up your muscles and improve your coordination quickly. The basic drumming techniques you'll end up using during this practice will be (Shawley, 2020):

- **singles**, where you strike your drum (the Pilates ball) with just your right or left hand

- **alternating singles**, where you alternate between your left and right hands as you strike the ball

- **doubles**, where you strike the ball with both sticks at the same time

- **bucket clicks**, where you strike the bucket the ball is standing on instead

- **drumming it out**, where you drum as fast as you possibly can

- **freestyling it**, where you drum however you'd like

Again, a good warm-up session will have you create all sorts of patterns with these moves and techniques, and may even have you add in some clicks, clacks, and taps to get you to move your entire body.

Stretching and Mobility Drills

Rhythm sticks can be a great tool to incorporate into your stretching and mobility skills, especially since they increase your reach. A 10-minute warm-up session should ideally be followed up with 5 minutes of stretching. Some basic stretches that you can incorporate your rhythm sticks into are (Mayo Clinic Staff, 2022):

- **hamstring stretches**, where you lie down on your back, raise your right leg up into the air while keeping the other one straight on the ground, and reach up with your left hand, trying to touch the tip of your rhythm stick to your flexed toes, then repeat on the other side

- **hip flexor stretches**, where you hold your sticks in both hands, kneel on your right knee, ideally on something soft like a yoga mat, place your other knee in front of you, place your left hand on your left leg, still holding the stick, keeping your other hand next to you, and hold the pose for 30 seconds

- **toe touches**, where you either keep your feet together and lean down to touch your rhythm sticks to your toes, or stand with your feet hip-width apart and lean down to touch your left toes with the stick in your right hand and your right toes with the stick in your left hand

- **over-the-shoulder stretches**, where you stand with your feet hip-width apart, place your left hand on your hip and reach up and over your head with your right hand, pointing toward the left with your stick, hold the pose for 30 seconds, and then do the same on the other side

- **wrist rotations**, where you stretch your left arm in front of you while keeping your stick perpendicular to the ground, tighten your arm, and move your wrist in a circular motion, before doing the same with your other hand and wrist

- **reach-ups**, where you grab a stick with one hand at each end and hold it horizontal to the ground, before raising it over your head and pushing up, without going on to your tiptoes

- **hip side stretches**, where you hold your sticks perpendicular to the ground and in front of your chest, tucking your elbows in close to your body, and rotate your upper body slowly to the left to stretch your side, and then slowly to the right, doing 10 repeats of this movement

These are just some examples of the kinds of stretches you can do with rhythm sticks. There are, however, many more. Of course, just because you're at a rhythm sticks cardio class or session doesn't mean you have to do all your stretches with sticks. You can throw some regular ones in there as well, like neck stretches, quadriceps stretches, and calf stretches. This way, you can make sure that all your muscle groups are properly prepared for your exercise round.

Chapter 4:

Essential Techniques for Rhythm Sticks Cardio

Assuming you have warmed up properly and followed up your warm-up exercises with some basic stretching moves, you are now ready to get started with rhythm sticks cardio. Before you can go deeply into the very cool choreographies, strength and balance exercises, and advanced rhythm sticks techniques, you'll first have to get your posture and grip just right. Maintaining the right posture in exercise is vital because it helps you to truly reap the benefits your workout has to offer you, and prevents you from injuring yourself (*Why Posture Matters*, 2017). It also allows you to execute the movements you're going to be doing correctly. Nailing the right posture, alignment, and grip when doing rhythm sticks cardio means being able to quickly master the basic striking techniques you'll be using, establish a steady rhythm and flow, and build on what you've learned to use even more complicated and, thus, more fun techniques and choreographies. So, what exactly does having the right grip and posture mean in rhythm sticks cardio? Let's find out!

Grip and Posture Alignment

In rhythm sticks cardio, grip refers to how you grasp the sticks that you are holding. A lot of us have the tendency to grip things really hard when we're working out, especially when we're doing something fast paced. This, however, is the wrong thing to do. Gripping your rhythm sticks too tightly is a bad idea because it locks your wrists in. This makes your wrists absorb more of the impact of any strikes, taps, and claps, thereby increasing your chance of injuring yourself. What you want to do instead is to grip your rhythm sticks loosely. You don't want your grip to be too loose, of course, lest your sticks go flying out of your hands. There is a delicate balance to strike here, one that you may be familiar with if you've ever played tennis, pickleball, table tennis, or something of the sort.

To strike this balance, you have to grip your sticks between your thumb and the first joint along your index finger. You'll know you've gripped your sticks correctly if your fingers are making the "okay" sign. Once they are, you can wrap your remaining fingers around your sticks. At this point, your grip should be firm but gentle. You can test whether or not this is the case by wiggling the sticks in your hand when they're tucked in between your index finger and your thumb. The sticks should have some range of movement there.

One thing you absolutely should not do is to extend your index finger so that it's resting along the stick. While this might feel comfortable to you, it will eventually result in one of your or your partner's sticks crash-landing on your finger, which will hurt at best and fracture at worst.

How about your posture, then? Well, you want to keep your back straight, your shoulders back, and your abdominal muscles engaged regardless of whether you're sitting down or standing up during your exercises. Your shoulders should also be relaxed and down. Meanwhile, your chin should be in line with your neck and your knees should not be locked. If you're standing up, your feet should be hip-width apart. If you're participating in cardio drumming while standing, you should adopt a slight squatting pose before your drum, so you can keep your core muscles engaged. If you're sitting down for a round of cardio drumming, then the ball you're going to be drumming on should be about chest level for you. That way, you won't have to overreach. The ball in question should be sitting on a bucket that it won't fall out of while you're drumming, and you'll also need to make sure the bucket isn't at risk of slipping around.

Basic Striking Techniques

There are a number of basic striking techniques you'll have to learn when you first get into rhythm sticks cardio. You'll recall some of these from your warm-up exercises, like L taps, R taps, clicks, and claps. There are many more on top of these, though. You'll be able to move onto these once you learn what taps, claps, and the like are. The remaining basic striking techniques that you will be practicing in your first few lessons are:

- **side clicks**, which will have you hit the sides of your ball at the same time

- **alternating bucket clicks**, where you alternate striking the bucket with your left, then right hand

- **floor taps**, where you strike the ground with both your sticks at the same time

- **alternating floor taps**, where you strike the ground with your rhythm sticks, while alternating between your left and right hands

- **front clicks**, where you hit your sticks together in front of your chest

- **overhead clicks**, where you strike your sticks together over your head

- **side clicks**, which have you strike your sticks together to one side

- **rainbow clicks**, where you start striking your sticks together on one side, click them together eight times while drawing an arching pattern that moves up and then down the way a rainbow would, and then repeating the same movement the opposite way, resulting in a grand total of 16 clicks and two rainbows

- **to the left**, which has you striking the ball or bucket of the individual to your left

- **to the right**, which has you striking the ball or bucket of the individual to your right

- **back to home**, which means going back to your own ball after striking the one next to yours

Once you have these basics down pat, you'll be able, mix, match, and combine them however you'd like, creating different patterns and unique choreographies in the process. Typically, each of these moves will be done in four counts, or for longer examples, like the rainbow clicks, in eight counts. This means that linking one move after the other can easily get your blood pumping. The more you master these moves, the easier it will be for you to switch between them, until you've developed a routine and can flow from one move to the next seamlessly.

Coordinating Rhythm and Movement

True to their name, rhythm sticks can really help you develop a sense of rhythm. They can do an even better job at this when they're paired with music, because then you'll be able to time your taps, clicks, and claps to the beat. This is why there are entire rhythm stick cardio choreographies for songs such as *We Will Rock You* and *Uptown Funk*. Those might be a little too advanced for beginners, though. A really great rhythm and movement exercise for newcomers to the sport, however, is rhythm sticks waltz. The waltz is an easy dance to couple with rhythm sticks because it has three beats per measure. You can match these beats both with the steps you take as you dance and with your taps, clicks, and claps.

The same goes for line dancing, funnily enough. A basic rhythm sticks line dancing routine can be:

- take a step to the left and do a front click

- take a step to the right and tap

- take a step to the left and tap

- do a turn

- do three taps on completing the turn

- slide to the side and do four overhead clicks

- slide to the other side and do another four overhead clicks

- repeat twice

Of course, a song usually lasts at least 2 minutes, so the more movement and taps you learn, the more complicated and varied the choreography you'll be able to create. It's essential, however, that you dedicate some time and energy to developing your own rhythm. To that end, you must start slowly and then gradually build up your speed. This way, you'll be able to make your workout more effective and enjoyable. You'll be able to truly pay attention to the music that's playing and slowly start to match your movements to it. It's only after you've mastered this skill that you can start adding variations to the routine you have developed.

Chapter 5:

Rhythm Sticks Cardio

Basics

You now know the basic techniques that you need to learn to get into rhythm sticks cardio, but what about the basic strategies? There are numerous strategies you can try out once you've mastered your basic techniques. Truthfully, these are all strategies that you will come across and be made to use in a regular rhythm sticks cardio session.

A typical rhythm sticks cardio session usually lasts about 30 minutes, not counting the warm-up and cool-down periods at the beginning and the end. They usually start out with slower patterns, then have you pick up speed. After you've gotten into the swing of things, however, they'll start throwing variations of speed into the mix. These will have you alternating between fast-paced drumming sequences and slower rhythms. As sessions go on, you might be introduced to different kinds of songs that you can experiment with, and you should do so since this will keep things fresh and exciting for you.

One very basic rhythm sticks cardio strategy is to incorporate full-body movements into your sessions and practices. Rhythm sticks cardio exercises are not exclusively an upper-body workout, and nor should they be. If you're engaged in this kind of workout, you should be moving your entire body, at least if you want to take advantage of all the benefits that cardio workouts have to offer you. This is why leg and core movements are a big part of rhythm sticks exercises. It's also why movements like lunges, squats, and steps need to be incorporated into your routine, even while you are drumming. That doesn't mean, however, that you should rush through the drumming movements. On the contrary, you should focus on making the movements as precise as you possibly can. To that end, your movements must be rhythmic but controlled. There should be no flailing movements or uncontrolled strikes.

Incorporating full-body movements into your rhythm sticks cardio session and focusing on precision over speed as you move will ultimately improve your overall stamina. The more of a flow you develop, the more moves you'll be able to add to your set and the more varied the choreographies you create will become. Over time, you'll be able to go for faster-paced songs too. To that end, choosing songs that are relatively slower paced is a good idea, at least in the beginning. With slower-paced songs, you'll typically be able to burn around 172–250 calories per hour. With faster-paced ones, like a good rock number, you'll be able to burn up to 600 calories per hour (Richardson, 2020). This is why a really good rhythm sticks cardio session can leave you as out of breath as if you had gone for a run, but again, you have to slowly work your way up to this. Otherwise, you'll end up pushing your body too hard and too fast, and you don't want to do that. So long as you keep this in mind, though, rhythm sticks cardio is a fantastic form of aerobic exercise.

Introduction to Rhythm Sticks Cardio Training

There are a lot of reasons why rhythm sticks cardio is a great option to consider for cardiovascular training. One key reason is that this workout can make you burn a couple of hundred calories in just 20 minutes. This makes sense when you think about it. I mean, there's a reason why some people have been able to lose as much as 70 pounds in 6 months through this cardio workout (Richardson, 2020). Another is that, thanks to those full-body movements that we talked about, like jumping, squats, dance moves, and steps, it gives your arms, legs, and core an active workout. That being the case, it shouldn't be surprising to hear that it lowers your blood pressure and keeps your stress hormones in check.

One unexpected benefit of rhythm sticks cardio is that it induces synchronous brain activity. Your brain has two separate hemispheres, as you know: the right one and the left one. These two hemispheres work on different frequencies and at different rates. Doing rhythm sticks cardio, however, activates both of them at the same time and helps them to coordinate with one another. This is especially true in cases where drumming is thrown into your routine. Rhythm sticks cardio, then, keeps both sides of your brain active and keeps your brain waves synchronized. As a rule, you want your brain waves to be synchronized because this calms your mind down significantly and increases your level of creativity. That rhythm sticks cardio increases the amount of alpha waves in your brain contributes to this significantly. Alpha waves are brain waves that generate a general feeling of well-being and relaxation, but about 30–40% of the population cannot generate alpha waves at all, at least not very easily (Conghalaigh, 2019). By doing rhythm sticks cardio, you can take yourself out of that 30–40% and enjoy a genuine state of relaxation.

Music and rhythm have been a part of human culture since pretty much the dawn of time. This is because they make us both happier and more self-aware. The same applies to rhythm sticks cardio, which uses sound and music exquisitely. Listening to the music around you and responding to it intuitively is a huge part of rhythm sticks cardio. This intuitive response system helps your brain to build strong neural connections between the movements you're performing and the beat you're listening to, which is why you become able to move faster and faster during sessions as time goes by.

One of the most important benefits that rhythm sticks cardio has to offer, at least for seniors, is that it helps reduce any pain they might be experiencing because of conditions like arthritis. Likewise, it can reduce any pain resulting from injuries they have sustained. There are two reasons for this. The first is that rhythm sticks cardio is really fun when you lose yourself in the rhythm of things—pun intended. The second is that it gets a great deal of endorphins to start pumping through your system, as most cardio workouts do. These endorphins effectively act as painkillers, which is why people struggling with chronic pain are often advised to exercise and move about. On top of this, though, rhythm sticks cardio has been found to be a good therapeutic method for people dealing with strokes and neurological diseases such as Parkinson's disease. It's even proven beneficial for people with attention deficit hyperactivity disorder (ADHD), since it does a lot to boost their level of concentration.

Benefits of Cardiovascular Exercise for Seniors

By now, it should be obvious that rhythm sticks cardio is incredibly beneficial for you. Some of these benefits are due to the unique nature of this form of exercise. Others stem from the very fact that it is cardio. One of the most obvious benefits that cardio has to offer seniors is that it strengthens their heart and cardiovascular system, as you know. This both enables them to prevent cardiovascular diseases and helps them to recover from them more quickly in the event that they do experience such a condition. This is partly due to the fact that cardio lowers your levels of bad cholesterol, which is otherwise known as low-density lipoprotein (LDL). At the same time, it raises your good cholesterol, which is known as high-density lipoprotein (HDL), to healthy heights.

As you might expect, cardio exercises are just as good for your respiratory system as they are for your heart.

This is why it's good for asthma, which is a fact that might be rather surprising to hear. You'd think that people who have asthma and other similar conditions should stay away from cardio, but you'd be wrong. In fact, medical professionals specifically recommend aerobic exercises like rhythm sticks cardio to people with asthma. This is because cardio expands these individuals' lung capacity. It expands everyone's lung capacity, really, so it's a good exercise model for anyone to pursue (Admin, 2020).

A lot of seniors curiously struggle with insomnia. Perhaps you do as well. If so, you'll be heartened to hear that cardio can help fix this too. Cardio is known to increase both the quality and duration of your sleep. The caveat with this is that you have to have finished your cardio exercise routine at least 2 hours before you go to bed. Otherwise, you'll unfortunately be struggling to fall asleep. A second caveat might be that you have to exercise regularly to truly reap this benefit.

Cardio has some interesting health benefits for your brain as well. For one, it increases your mental acuity and makes you think a lot more clearly than you otherwise could (Gomez-Pinilla & Hillman, 2013). Studies show that regular cardio exercise actually reduces your risk of developing conditions like Alzheimer's disease (Alzheimer's Association, n.d.). This is likely due to the curious connection that exists between Alzheimer's and heart disease. You see, it turns out that 80% of all individuals who have Alzheimer's also have some type of heart disease. Often, these are the kinds of heart disease where a lot of plaque builds up in your veins. These plaques then travel up to your brain via your bloodstream and cause some damage, somehow leading to Alzheimer's. Though it isn't entirely clear yet how this process works, one thing is obvious: By doing cardio exercises regularly, you can strengthen your heart, keep from developing heart disease, and thus protect yourself against mental decline and conditions like Alzheimer's disease and dementia.

You already know that regular exercise can increase your mobility and thus make you more independent, but did you know that regular cardio can improve your sense of balance too? Studies show that regular cardio workouts can improve your balance so much that they'll reduce your chance of experiencing some kind of fall by as much as 23% (Manor, 2019). Judging by all this, you can clearly see that cardio is absolutely essential for anyone who wants to lead a healthy, strong, and free lifestyle and age well.

Cardio Routines With Rhythm Sticks

"This is all well and good, but how do I do cardio workouts with rhythm sticks?" I can almost hear you asking. Truthfully, there are numerous cardio routines that you can try out. Some of these are full-on dance routines, which are incredibly fun and sure to work up a good sweat. These, though, will be covered in detail in the coming chapters. In the meantime, there are a number of other cardio routines you can and should try out. One strategy to adopt here might be to settle on two or three different routines and alternate between them every few days. That way, you can keep things from getting boring, if that's a concern for you, and ensure that you're working all your muscle groups. With this in mind, here are a couple of sample routines you can try with rhythm sticks:

- *The Four Minute Sticks Workout* (Runner Bean Health & Fitness, 2021):

  o Do 10 minutes of warm-up exercises and 5 minutes of stretching.

  o Stand with your feet wide apart.

  o Do 10 overhead clicks in time with the rhythm of whatever music you've put on.

  o Lower your hands to alternate sides six times (each) as you keep the beat.

  o Lower and raise both hands to your sides 10 times as you keep the beat.

  o Do 10 side clicks to the left as you keep the beat.

  o Do 10 side clicks to the right as you keep the beat.

  o Do 10 side clicks to the left as you keep the beat.

  o Do 10 side clicks to the right as you keep the beat.

  o Do 10 overhead clicks as you keep the beat.

- Alternate tapping the floor in front of you to the left and to the right, six times each, as you keep the beat. Clap the sticks together in front of your chest between each tap, rising from your crouch slightly.

- Grab your sticks in both hands so that they're horizontal to the ground and push them up over your head 12 times as you keep the beat while doing box steps (stepping to the four corners of an imaginary box). There should be one step per arm raise.

- Reverse the direction of the box steps and repeat another 12 times as you keep the beat.

- Do eight overhead clicks with single arms as you keep the beat.

- Do eight overhead clicks with both arms.

- Do six side clicks to the left as you keep the beat.

- Do six side clicks to the right as you keep the beat.

- Grab your sticks in both hands so that they're horizontal to the ground and push them up over your head 12 times as you keep the beat while doing box steps . There should be one step per arm raise.

- ○ Reverse the direction of the box steps and repeat another 12 times as you keep the beat.

- ○ Do six overhead clicks with single arms as you keep the beat.

- ○ Do six overhead clicks (or doubles) with both arms.

- ○ Do another six doubles while turning with each tap.

- ○ Do six floor taps in front of you, rising from your crouch slightly after you've tapped the ground to clap your sticks in front of your chest.

- ○ End with 10 overhead clicks as you keep the beat.

- ○ Do a 10-minute cool-down and a 5-minute stretching session.

- *The Forty Minute Sticks Workout* (Revelation Wellness, 2022)

  - ○ Do 10 minutes of warm-up exercises and 5 minutes of stretching.

  - ○ Start by doing 10 side steps.

  - ○ Add an upper body rotation, slowly punching out with one of your hands (which will be clutching your rhythm stick) to the opposite side as you go and raising the heel of your opposite foot off the ground each time.

- ○ Do 10 alternating reach-ups, your hands still clasping your rhythm sticks.

- ○ Do 10 reps of your upper body rotations and punches.

- ○ Start jogging slightly in place for 15 seconds.

- ○ Take three side steps to the left, do an overhead click, then take three side steps to the right, and do an overhead click. Repeat eight times in each direction.

- ○ Do eight side steps without moving from your spot, stepping back to your starting position each time, extending your arms forward as you step to the side.

- ○ Get into a slight squat position, holding your arms in front of you, keeping them bent at the elbows. Then start rotating to the sides from your knees, slowly punching out with the opposite hand with each turn. Return to your starting position after every rotation-punch, and repeat eight times on each side.

o   Do 10 alternating reach-ups, your hands still clasping your rhythm sticks.

o   Start marching in place and pick up the speed a bit. Keep going for 30 seconds.

o   Start jogging slightly in place for 15 seconds.

o   Take three side steps to the left, do an overhead click, then take three side steps to the right, and do another overhead click. Repeat eight times.

o   Slowly kick your legs up, each one in turn, keeping them below your waist line, clapping your sticks in front of your chest with every kick and opening your arms up to your sides after each kick, keeping your elbows bent. Do eight reps per leg.

o   Take a 30-second break.

o   Get into a slight squatting position and start shifting your weight from leg to leg. Keep going like that for 30 seconds.

o   Continue shifting your weight but start reaching down toward the ground with your sticks with each shift, then pulling your hands back to the sides of your hips. Keep going like that for 30 seconds.

- Stop swaying and start tapping the ground in front of you. Go for 30 seconds if you can.

- Do three taps on the ground and then three overhead clicks. Repeat this sequence four to eight times.

- Do three overhead clicks and reach for your left heel with your left stick after the third one, keeping your right arm up. Do three overhead clicks and then reach for your right heel, keeping your left arm up. Repeat this sequence six times.

- Do one overhead click, reach for your left heel, keeping your right arm up, then reach for your right heel, keeping your left arm up, and do another overhead click. Repeat six times.

- Do eight floor taps.

- Do eight overhead clicks.

- Do one overhead click, reach for your left heel, keeping your right arm up, then reach for your right heel, keeping your left arm up, and do another overhead click. Repeat six times.

- Take a 20-second break.

- Repeat the entire sequence from the beginning twice.

- End with a 10-minute cool-down session and a 5-minute stretching session.

Chapter 6:

Rhythm Sticks Strength

and Balance Training

While rhythm sticks are great for cardio, that's not the only thing they can be used for. They can also be incorporated into strength and balance exercises, which are very necessary for seniors' general health and well-being, just as cardio workouts are. Before we go into why seniors need these things, though, let's properly establish what they are. Strength training, alternatively known as resistance training or weight training, is a form of exercise that is designed to work and strengthen the various muscle groups of your body (Iliades, 2018). It accomplishes this by having you use free weights such as dumbbells, weight machines if you happen to be in the gym, or your own body weight. The idea here is to overload your muscles, so that they are forced to adapt to the new conditions they are facing and, thus, get stronger.

Balance training, meanwhile, is a kind of workout method that seeks to improve your stance, gait, and posture, thereby improving your balance, as the name indicates. Balance training can be incredibly important for seniors given their propensity for experiencing falls and how dangerous this can be for them. That much should be clear. What's likely not as clear is why strength training is important and necessary for seniors. So, before we dive into how you can incorporate rhythm sticks into your strength-training exercises—something that sounds like it's hard to do seeing as rhythm sticks don't weigh all that much—let's take a look at why you need to make this type of workout a part of your everyday life in the first place (Watson, 2014).

Importance of Strength and Balance Training for Seniors

While a lot of people do work out these days, they often go for things like cardio over strength training. This is problematic because strength training is absolutely vital if you want to live a long life and age well. This doesn't mean you should choose strength training over cardio workouts, of course. What you should do instead is to do both. You don't necessarily have to do cardio and strength training on the same days. You can squeeze your strength-training sessions in on days where you're not doing cardio workouts. Ideally, seniors should be doing strength training once or twice a week.

The primary reason you want to do this is that strength training prevents the muscle mass loss that comes with aging (Cleveland Clinic, 2019). This muscle loss is known as sarcopenia and it is a natural phenomenon. It is also an eminently debilitating one, enough to reduce your mobility, strength, stamina, and independence significantly. The reason you experience sarcopenia has to do with the neurological signals your brain sends regarding muscle growth. There are two types of muscle growth signals: One tells your muscles to reduce their size, while the other tells them to increase it. When you turn 50, your brain starts sending the former message out far more often than it does the latter. Your body obeys the order it is being given, hence the shrinkage. This situation, though, is reversible, so long as you are willing to lead a more active lifestyle and do some strength training.

The prevention of muscle loss isn't the only benefit strength training has to offer you. There are many others, such as the prevention of health conditions like obesity and even heart conditions, if recent studies are anything to go by (Mcleod et al., 2019). You're probably thinking that cardio is more likely to help you with obesity and other weight-related conditions than strength training. You'll be surprised to learn, then, that your supposition is incorrect. While cardio can and does help with weight loss, strength training is no less effective at it. Strength training boosts your metabolism, making you burn a lot more calories a lot faster. Coupled with cardio exercises, this can make you shed a lot of pounds incredibly rapidly, especially since your body continues burning through calories after you're done with your strength-training routine. Strength training also makes you start consuming a lot more oxygen after your workouts than before. This also boosts your weight-loss efforts.

One side effect of building muscle mass is that it keeps you burning calories, even while you're sleeping. As interesting as that is, though, the most fascinating benefit that strength training has to offer, by far, is that it actually helps you to live longer. According to one study, strength training extends your life span and reduces your mortality rate, even when you catch a major, noncommunicable disease (Momma et al., 2022). This, mind you, isn't a benefit that cardio can offer you and is only applicable to strength training. On top of that, strength training helps you live better by making it easier for you to manage any chronic conditions you may have, like HIV, any neuromuscular disorders, and even certain types of cancer (Beavers et al., 2017). Simultaneously, it improves your glucose levels, which is great news for people with type 2 diabetes and a prime reason why these individuals should be prioritizing strength training.

As if those benefits weren't enough, strength training increases your ability to move around a little more than cardio can too. This is because strength training primarily involves movements like lifting, pulling, and pushing things. In other words, they're functional movements that you will have to perform in your everyday life. So, the more you work the muscles you need to perform these movements, the stronger those muscles will become and the more easily and freely you'll be able to go about your daily business.

One last benefit this training method has to offer is that it boosts your energy levels and improves your mood and, therefore, your mental health. Several studies have found that strength training tamps down the symptoms of depression. Of course, it gives you a burst of endorphins too, much like cardio, making you feel better overall (Bennington-Castro, 2022).

What about balance training, then? Your sense of balance is likely not something you think about often, at least not until you lose your balance and find yourself crash-landing on the ground. Yet balance is an essential part of your everyday life. You rely on it when you're sitting down or getting up from the couch. You use it when walking from one place to another and when you're reaching for something on a high shelf. Put simply, your balance is something you need and use all of the time. If you want your sense of balance to remain, you need your muscles to stay strong. You also need to test and improve your balance through various specific, targeted exercises. Hence, balance training.

Balance training won't just improve your balance. It will improve your reflexes and reaction times too, both of which will be very important if and when you trip and fall. Simultaneously, balance training can improve your overall coordination. Being coordinated isn't just good for preventing falls; it's good for preventing injuries when you fall as well. Part of the reason people get injured when they fall is that they simply crash down onto the ground. This isn't what you want to do. Instead, you want to roll with the fall. That probably doesn't make much sense when put like that, so picture this scenario: You're walking down the road and someone pushes you for some reason. You're unable to stop your fall and the ground is fast approaching. You can do one of two things in this case: Either you can fall on your face and really hurt something, or you can go with the trajectory of the fall, roll your body as much as possible, and have a softer part of your body, like the side of your arm, absorb most of the impact. In which case would you be injured worse, the former or the latter? The answer to that question is of course "the latter," and that's what you can ensure happens by doing balance training.

Strength and Balance Exercises With Rhythm Sticks

Based on all of this, the real question isn't whether or not you should be doing strength and balance straining; the real question is how you can incorporate your rhythm sticks into your strength and balance exercises. There are many ways in which you can do this. Some examples include:

- **Squats:** Squats are a move you will often have to perform in your rhythm sticks cardio classes and sessions. They're actually a strength-training move because they make you lift and use your own body weight. It's the kind of move that engages your abdominal and lower-body muscles and gives them a proper workout. To perform a squat, stand with your feet shoulder-width apart and hold your arms in front of your chest. Your hands will, naturally, be holding your rhythm sticks. That done, you will bend at the hips and start lowering your behind as if you were going to sit down on an invisible chair. You will keep lowering yourself until your knees are bent at a 90-degree angle. Once you're in that position, you can either clap your rhythm sticks together or tap them against the Pilates-ball-turned-drum that's stationed before you. Then you can rise back up to your original position (Ollie, 2021).

- **Knee thrusters:** Stand with your feet a little farther than shoulder-width apart and turn both your feet to the left. Make sure that your hips are facing the same direction as your feet. This will drop you down into a shallow lunge, with your knees slightly bent. Grab your rhythm sticks in both hands, holding them by the ends so that they are parallel to the ground. Keep your rhythm sticks in front of your chest, slowly raise your front knee up, and try to touch it to your rhythm sticks. Try not to lower your hands down in the process. Then, lower your foot down, and repeat for 1 minute. Turn to the other side and repeat the same movements with your other knee for another minute (Freytag, 2022).

- **Lunges:** Stand with your feet hip-width apart and hold your arms in front of your chest, with your rhythm sticks in your hands. Take one step back with your right foot but leave your left foot where it is. Slowly bend your back knee and lower it to the ground. As you do, raise your hands up and do an overhead click when you stop. Slowly return to your original position and do eight reps. Then switch legs and do the same thing another eight times.

- **Squat curl knee lifts:** Grab your rhythm sticks and drop into your regular squat position. Keep your arms extended to your sides and drop your weight onto your heels. Push up on your heels as you rise back to a standing position, squeezing your leg muscles as you go. Slowly, raise your left knee toward your chest once you're standing, then curl your rhythm sticks up to your chest and clap them together in front of you, keeping your elbows bent. Slowly put your foot back down, lower your arms to their starting position, and drop back down to a squat. Do eight reps, then eight more with your other knee.

- **Sit-ups:** Lie down on a comfortable surface such as a yoga mat and extend your arms over your head, holding a rhythm stick in each hand. Keep your arms and legs long and flex your feet. Take a deep breath and lift your arms up. As you do, start curling your chin into your chest, then roll your whole torso up. Clap your sticks together overhead when you're sitting up to perform an overhead clap, then keep rolling forward. Keep your abs engaged the whole time and reach for your toes with your sticks, though it's alright if they stretch beyond your toes. Once you've made contact with your toes, exhale and slowly roll back down, a vertebra at a time, and return to your starting position. Do eight reps.

- **Calf raises:** Stand with your feet close together and hold your arms in front of and close to your chest, with a rhythm stick in each hand. Slowly rise up onto your toes and extend your arms up and over your head if you can. Once you're on your tiptoes, clap your rhythm sticks together. If you're unable to raise your hands above your head, extend them slightly in front of you as you rise onto your tiptoes and clap your sticks together there. Then, slowly lower yourself back down to your heels and return your hands to their original positions. Do eight reps (*Easy Leg Exercises for Seniors*, 2021).

- **Marching in place:** Stand with your feet close together and hold your rhythm sticks in front of your chest, shoulder-width apart. Then, lift your left knee as high as you can. Once you've hit the highest point you can go, clap your rhythm sticks together, lower your knee, and raise your other knee up to your chest. Clap your sticks together again. If you're struggling with balance, only do one clap per two knee lifts. Keep going in this fashion until you've done 20 to 25 reps.

- **Single leg stand:** Stand with your feet together, your back straight, and your arms at your sides, holding a rhythm stick in each hand. Slowly raise your right hand above your head, then raise your left foot until your knee is perpendicular. Stay in this position for 10 to 15 seconds. If this proves a little too challenging for you, hold out both your hands in front of you, holding your rhythm sticks, and slowly raise your left foot. Clap your rhythm sticks in front of you 10 to 15 times, then lower your foot down to its original position. Switch legs and do the same thing for the same amount of time.

- **Step-ups:** Take a box or a step and take up position behind it, with your rhythm sticks in your hands. Carefully step onto the box or step with just one leg and do three claps in front of you with your rhythm sticks. Then, slowly lift the foot that's on the step and rotate your ankle in the air five to seven times. Gently place it down, take a step back, and repeat the same movements with your other foot. Do eight reps.

Modifications and Progressions for Different Fitness Levels

Some of the strength- and balance-training movements we've covered here may be a little too difficult for you at your current fitness level. Perhaps they are a little too advanced for you. Perhaps you have other considerations that must be kept in mind. The good news is that this doesn't mean you have to forgo strength-training exercises. Instead, you can modify them to suit your needs, as follows:

- **Modified squats** (Young, 2021a):

    - **The narrow squat:** Stand with your feet hip-width apart and your toes pointing forward. Keep your arms bent at your sides. Then push your hips back and start bending your knees, going down only as far as is comfortable and manageable for you. Bring your hands together in front of your chest and clap your rhythm sticks when you stop, then slowly rise back up and reposition your arms at your sides.

- The alternating side squat: Keep your feet close together this time and keep your arms slightly bent at your sides. Take a step to your right with your right foot, but don't move your left foot, making sure that your toes point forward as they land. Push your hips back to squat. Go as low as is comfortable for you and clap your sticks together when you stop. Then rise back to your feet, pushing up from your heels as you go, and return to your original position. Repeat the same movement with your left foot and side.

- **Modified lunges** (Young, 2021b):

  - **The seated lunge squeeze:** Sit down sideways on a chair, with your feet planted firmly on the ground. Bend your outside knee toward the ground, keeping your weight on the chair. Keep your back straight, take a deep breath, and squeeze your glutes. As you do so, raise your arms over your head to do an overhead click with your sticks. Exhale and release the tension while you lower your arms down to chest level. Repeat this move for a total of eight times, before sitting the opposite way in your chair and doing the same with your opposite leg for another eight reps.

○ **Modified reverse lunge:** Stand behind a sturdy chair and place a hand on its back for support. Hold one rhythm stick in your other, free hand, which will be held in front of your chest. Shift your weight to one foot, raise your other knee up, and place your toes on the ground behind you. Once you're feeling well-balanced, shift your weight to your front foot and bend your knees so you drop down into a lunge. Keeping your back straight, raise your stick-wielding hand above your head as you go. Exhale as you rise back up and lower your hand back to chest level. Do eight reps, before turning around and repeating the move with your other foot in front.

- **Modified seated roll-ups:** Sit down on a sturdy chair and extend your legs forward before you. Flex your feet so that your toes are pointing up to the ceiling. Keep your back straight and extend your arms in front of you, keeping hold of one rhythm stick in each hand. Start curling forward from your chin and breathe out as you roll your torso over your legs, reaching for your toes. When you get to the point where you can't roll any farther, clap your sticks together underneath your legs and take a breath as you roll back up to your starting position, one vertebra at a time. Do eight reps (Bedosky, 2022).

- **Modified seated leg raises:** Sit in a sturdy chair and extend your right leg in front of you with your toes flexed up to the ceiling, keeping the other leg bent with your foot planted firmly on the ground. Grab hold of the side of your chair with your right hand. Your left hand should be holding a rhythm stick. Next, raise your extended foot up so that it becomes horizontal to, and about a foot off, the ground. Extend your left hand and point at your toes with the rhythm stick you are holding. Slowly lower both your arm and your leg. Complete eight reps, then extend your other leg, switch hands, and repeat the movement another eight times.

Chapter 7:

Cardio Dance Routines

With Rhythm Sticks

Now that you're acquainted with the various moves you can perform with rhythm sticks, let's take a look at the dance routines you can incorporate them into. Rhythm sticks cardio relies heavily on music and dance and typically creates a variety of dance numbers that prove to be excellent cardio workouts. As a beginner, you should choose a song with a slower kind of rhythm to choreograph your first dance routine to. After a while, meaning after your endurance levels have gone up a bit and you've mastered the basic moves, you can go for faster, more upbeat numbers.

Cardio dance routines with rhythm sticks are considered to be a form of dance fitness. They are a type of workout where the focus isn't on the choreography or the excellence of your pirouette. Rather, it's on doing your best to follow your instructor, working up a sweat, getting your heart rate elevated, and having fun. The great thing about this type of dance is that other exercise techniques, such as strength-training and balance-training moves can easily be worked into it.

Exploring Dance-Based Cardio Workouts

Cardio dance workouts have specific benefits to offer in and of themselves and come in an array of styles. Activities like Zumba, for instance, definitely count as cardio dance, as do cardio drumming and cardio dancing with rhythm sticks, which are admittedly more musical and, well, rhythmic than things like Zumba. After all, you have to match the beat that you're hearing with the percussive instruments that you're holding. A lot of dance cardio classes last around 45 minutes, not counting your warm-up and cool-down sessions. A cardio dance session that's only 20 minutes long will still be incredibly effective, as you no doubt know by now. Some cardio dances can be heavily choreographed, whereas others can be more freestyle. Given rhythm sticks cardio's emphasis on beat and rhythm, it tends to be more choreography heavy, even if said choreography mostly makes use of steps and various fitness moves such as lunges and squats.

The best thing about dance cardio workouts—aside from all the health benefits, of course—is that they can be very social but also very conducive to solo, at-home practice. Once you've nailed a choreography, you can easily blast the music at home and practice there to your heart's content. Most people prefer going to actual dance classes, since getting into the swing of things is easier when you're surrounded by other dancers, but having the option to stay at home can be rather appealing, especially in the post-pandemic world.

So, what kinds of moves can you expect to see in a typical rhythm sticks cardio choreography? The short answer to that question is "lots." The long answer includes:

- **Jumping jacks**, which involve standing up with your feet hip-width apart and your arms at your sides, then bending your knees slightly and jumping into the air, spreading your feet to shoulder-width apart as you jump. While jumping, stretch your hands over your head and perform an overhead clap with your rhythm sticks, before landing back down on the ground and falling into your starting position (*How to Do a Jumping Jack*, 2019).

- **Booty pops**, which require standing with your feet shoulder-width apart, leaning forward with your upper body so that you form a 45-degree angle. Keeping your weight on your toes, you then swivel your hips from side to side while keeping your hands in front of you and clapping your rhythm sticks either in front of you or to the sides, if you'd prefer (Horvath-Krol, 2020).

- **Side shuffles**, where you start by keeping your feet a little wider than hip-width apart while pointing both your toes and knees forward. Follow that up by taking a couple of really quick steps to the left, tapping your left foot with your left rhythm stick, then doing the same in the other direction with your right hand and foot, all while remaining in a light squat position, keeping your back straight and looking straight ahead (Spotebi, 2015).

- **Single-leg hip hikes**, where you keep your feet together and your hands to the sides before shifting your weight to one foot and raising your other foot slightly off the floor. Then, keeping your grounded foot straight, bend your upper body slightly to the side and over the hip of the leg whose foot is on the floor, before returning to your original position and repeating the same movement with your other leg and side (Falk, 2022).

- **Thrusters**, which involve dropping down into a squat, then raising your arms overhead to clap your rhythm sticks together there, making sure that they return to their position over your shoulders after every clap with your biceps pressing against your ears.

- **Toe-taps**, where you start lightly—though you can pick up the speed if you'd like—jogging in place behind an object such as a step, tapping the toes of your left and right feet on it alternately.

- **Lateral shuffles**, which have you stand with your feet hip-width apart, dispersing your weight evenly and tightening your abdominal muscles. Push off from your left foot, then shuffle to the right five times, making sure that your chest remains in line with your knees with each move, before repeating the same move in the opposite direction.

Moves like squats and lunges, which you already know how to do, also sneak their way into rhythm sticks cardio dance routines on a regular basis, which is good news because studies show that such exercises significantly strengthen your lungs and your heart (Falk, 2022). Thanks to all this, dance cardio can offer you a great many benefits. For starters, it improves both your flexibility and your agility. More specifically, it improves your joint, hip, and spinal flexibility, which is important for older adults because the more flexible these parts of your body are, the less likely you will be to strain, fracture, or otherwise injure them (Alricsson & Werner, 2004).

Your memory and cognitive capabilities are also very important as you age. You want to ensure that your faculties are in good, strong condition, after all. Cardio dance, it turns out, can be uniquely good for this, as it can prevent cognitive decline because new neural pathways form in your brain as you perform the various movements associated with your choreography. The more new movements you add into the mix, the more neural pathways will form, and the more you'll be protected against cognitive decline. This makes cardio dance even more effective in preventing diseases such as Alzheimer's than other cardio workouts (Merom et al., 2016).

Choreographed Rhythm Sticks Dance Routines

There are a vast number of choreographed rhythm sticks dance routines out there, if we're being honest. So, you might understandably be confused as to where to start and which one to choose. That being the case, here are a couple of samples that you might consider trying out:

- Jennifer Lopez's *Dance Again* (Ramos, 2020):

  - Do 15 overhead clicks with alternating heel and toe taps.

  - Do 10 box steps with front clicks.

  - Jump to the back, squat, and tap the ground.

  - Jump back to the front, squat, and tap the ground in front of you with both hands.

  - Jump and take a step forward and back and tap the ground next to your front foot with one hand.

  - Jump and take a reverse step backward and forward, and tap the ground next to your front foot with one hand.

  - Do a side shuffle to the left, clapping your rhythm sticks in front of you as you go.

  - Do a side shuffle to the right, clapping your rhythm sticks in front of you as you go.

  - Tap the ground in front of you.

  - Do three rapid overhead claps.

- Do a side shuffle to the right, clapping your rhythm sticks in front of you as you go.

- Do a side shuffle to the left, clapping your rhythm sticks in front of you as you go.

- Slide to the left and do an overhead click, then tap the ground in front of you.

- Do five overhead claps.

- Slide to the right and do an overhead click, then tap the ground in front of you.

- Slide to the left and do an overhead click, then tap the ground in front of you.

- Do five overhead claps.

- Do eight overhead claps with alternating toe and heel taps.

- Do 10 box steps with front clicks.

- Jump back to the front, squat, and tap the ground in front of you.

- Jump and take a step forward and back, and tap the ground next to your front foot.

- Do a side shuffle to the left, clicking your rhythm sticks in front of you as you go.

- Do a side shuffle to the right, clicking your rhythm sticks in front of you as you go.

- Take three steps back and do five rapid overhead claps.

- Do a side shuffle to the right, clicking your rhythm sticks in front of you as you go.

- Do a side shuffle to the left, clicking your rhythm sticks in front of you as you go.

- Take three steps forward and tap the ground in front of you with both hands.

- Slide to the right and clap, then tap the ground in front of you.

- Do five claps.

- Slide to the left and clap, then tap the ground in front of you.

- Do five claps in front of you.

- Slide to the right and clap, then tap the ground in front of you.

- Do five claps.

- Slide to the left and clap, then tap the ground in front of you.

  - Do five claps.

- Queen's *We Will Rock You* (Martinez, 2017)

  - Do two front and two overhead claps, keeping to the initial rhythm and bending your knees slightly as you do the front claps. Repeat until the initial rhythmic part of the song is over.

  - Do slight lateral, alternating kicks, pointing at your rising and flexing toes each time with your rhythm sticks.

  - Do two front and two overhead claps, keeping to the initial rhythm and bending your knees slightly as you do the front claps. Repeat until the rhythmic part of the song is over.

  - Do slight lateral, alternating kicks, pointing at your rising and flexing toes each time with your rhythm sticks.

  - Do two front and two overhead claps, keeping to the initial rhythm and bending your knees slightly as you do the front claps. Repeat twice.

  - Raise your right heel up behind you, twisting your knee so that your foot is slightly to the side and tap it twice with your right rhythm stick. Lower your foot back down, then do two overhead claps before raising your left heel up behind you, twisting your knee so that your foot is slightly to the side and tapping it twice with your rhythm stick.

○ Do slight lateral, alternating kicks, pointing at your rising and flexing toes each time with your rhythm sticks.

○ Do two front and two overhead claps, keeping to the initial rhythm and bending your knees slightly as you do the front claps. Repeat twice.

○ Do slight lateral, alternating kicks, pointing at your rising and flexing toes each time with your rhythm sticks.

○ Keeping your knees slightly bent, lower your right rhythm stick down to your right knee, then your left rhythm stick to your left knee, and then raise them back up over your head. Do eight reps of this.

○ Do slight lateral, alternating kicks, pointing at your rising and flexing toes each time with your rhythm sticks.

○ Do two front and two overhead claps, keeping to the initial rhythm and bending your knees slightly as you do the front claps. Repeat twice.

- Do slight lateral, alternating kicks, pointing at your rising and flexing toes each time with your rhythm sticks.

  - Do two front and two overhead claps, keeping to the initial rhythm and bending your knees slightly as you do the front claps. Repeat twice.

  - Do slight lateral, alternating kicks, pointing at your rising and flexing toes each time with your rhythm sticks.

  - Do two front and two overhead claps, keeping to the initial rhythm and bending your knees slightly as you do the front claps. Repeat twice.

  - Step out to your right with your right foot and do two clicks to your right. Step back to your original position and do two overhead claps. Then, step to your left side with your left foot, then do two clicks there. Step back to your original position. Keep going until the music ends.

- Mark Ronson's *Uptown Funk* (Condran, 2019):

  - Do four lateral shuffles going from left to right, clicking your rhythm sticks in front of you for each one.

  - Do another four lateral shuffles going from left to right, performing overhead clicks as you go.

- Do four lateral shuffles going from left to right, clicking your rhythm sticks in front of you for each one.

- Do four lateral shuffles going from left to right, performing overhead clicks as you go.

- Do eight lateral, alternating kicks, raising your rhythm sticks over your head (without tapping them) with each kick, and slightly lowering them as you move your leg back to its original position.

- Hold out one rhythm stick directly before you in your right hand and sweep it toward the right, while keeping your other hand hanging by your side. Drop your right hand to your side and do the same move with your left hand. Repeat eight times.

- Shuffle your feet and grab your rhythm sticks in the middle. One at a time, roll them from your chest to your waist like you're striking a drum there four times, then brush your shoulders with the sticks, twice on each side. Repeat this sequence four times.

- Keeping your feet together, jump from right to left to right and do an overhead clap, then jump from left to right to left and do an overhead clap. Repeat twice.

- Jog in place for 30 seconds.

- Do one jumping jack and land with your feet wide apart.

- Take a big side step to the right, land in a slight squat, and swish your knees while drawing large figure-eights with your sticks.

- Take a big side step to the left, land in a slight squat, and swish your knees while drawing large figure-eights with your sticks.

- Take a big side step to the right, land in a slight squat, and swish your knees while drawing large figure-eights with your sticks.

- Take a big side step to the left, land in a slight squat, and swish your knees while drawing large figure-eights with your sticks.

- Reach up with your rhythm sticks, reach to the sides, and crouch to tap the ground twice. Repeat thrice more.

- Hold your rhythm sticks from the center, keeping them parallel to the ground. Then turn them so they're perpendicular and move the right over the left as if you're pouring water into the left one from the right. Do the same with the left over the right. Lower your right stick to your side and pretend to take a drink of water from the left one, then do the reverse. Repeat four times.

o   Hold your rhythm sticks from the center and move your arms diagonally, one hand raising up to point at 3 o'clock, the other pointing down at 7 o'clock, by your side, opening up your chest as you go. Switch the position of your hands and repeat the movements eight times, pointing your toes alternately in and out with each movement.

o   Shuffle your feet and grab your rhythm sticks in the middle. One at a time, roll them from your chest to your waist like you're striking a drum there four times, then brush your shoulders with them, twice on each side. Repeat this sequence four times.

o   Keeping your feet together, jump from right to left to right and do an overhead clap, then jump from left to right to left and do an overhead clap. Repeat twice.

o   Jog in place for 30 seconds.

o   Take a big side step to the right, land in a slight squat, and swish your knees while drawing large figure-eights with your sticks.

o   Take a big side step to the left, land in a slight squat, and swish your knees while drawing large figure-eights with your sticks.

o   Squat down and tap your rhythm sticks twice on the ground before raising them over your head and rising back up, pushing the sticks out to your sides at chest level, and then sinking back down to tap the ground again. Repeat thrice.

o   March in place doing overhead presses with your rhythm sticks for 30 seconds.

o   Do alternating lateral kicks, punching out with the same side hand as you go. Repeat four times per side.

o   Take a big side step to the right, land in a slight squat, and swish your knees while drawing large figure-eights with your sticks.

o   Take a big side step to the left, land in a slight squat, and swish your knees while drawing large figure-eights with your sticks.

o   Squat down and tap your rhythm sticks twice on the ground before raising them over your head and rising back up. Then push your arms out to your sides at chest level, before sinking back down to tap the ground again. Repeat thrice.

- o Take three small steps to the left and march in place, doing overhead presses with your rhythm sticks, for 30 seconds.

- o Shuffle to the right, taking five steps and keeping your rhythm sticks in front of your chest with your elbows bent, pushing out with each step. Switch directions and repeat.

- o March in place, doing overhead presses with your rhythm sticks, for 30 seconds.

- o Jump from side to side, keeping your feet close together, as you wave your rhythm sticks over your head with each move.

- o End with a jumping jack and pose.

Building Coordination and Memory Skills

Dance cardio with rhythm sticks requires having two specific skills: coordination and memory. Your coordination is your ability to use your various body parts together in harmony. Suddenly changing the direction you are walking in is something that requires some degree of coordination, for example. Coordination allows you to be more agile in your movements and adjust to changes quickly. Once you've mastered a move, it helps you to perform it perfectly and then follow it up with another, equally perfect move. Put simply, coordination is what enables you to execute different moves with different parts of your body at the same time and create a genuine flow between the sequences in your choreography.

Now, you might be thinking that some people are just more naturally coordinated than others. This isn't necessarily the case. Coordination is actually one of those skills that you can improve upon with some practice, patience, and the help of some specific exercises. Some examples of such exercises might be (Fatima, 2023):

- **Heel-to-toe walking**, where you place your right foot directly in front of your left foot, your right heel touching your left toes, then place your left foot directly in front of your right foot with your left heel touching your right toes, and keep walking in that manner in a completely straight line. This exercise will strengthen your calf and ankle muscles specifically, so long as you start by placing your weight on your heels and then shifting it to your toes as you walk, and take at least 20 steps. It can be done while you hold your rhythm sticks in your hands, with your arms at your sides for balance.

- **Marching in place**, for which you'll need to stand with your back straight and start by lifting your right knee as high as possible, then lowering it. Follow it up by raising your left knee as high as possible. Keep going like that, raising your knees a minimum of 20 times to strengthen your lower-body muscles including your quadriceps, hip flexors, calves, hamstrings, and tibialis anterior. You can clap your rhythm sticks in front of you each time you raise a knee and establish a rhythm if you'd like.

- **Single limb stance with arm extensions**, where you stand with your feet together, your back straight, and your arms at your sides. Slowly raise your right foot off the ground as you raise your left hand to the ceiling. Point with your raised hand to the ceiling. Hold that position for about 10 seconds, then lower both your arm and your leg, and assume the same position with your other arm and leg. Do this about 10 times for each arm/leg combination. In doing so, you will strengthen your core and lower-body muscles and improve your coordination, as well as your sense of balance.

- **Clock reaches**, where you pretend you are standing at the very center of a clock, with 6 o'clock in front of you and 12 o'clock behind you. You then slowly raise your right hand and arm into the air and point at 12 o'clock. After holding that pose for a few seconds, point to 3 o'clock with just your raised arm. Then, trace a path back to 6 o'clock and, finally, end by pointing at 3 o'clock, then 12 o'clock, before lowering both your arm and leg. You then repeat the same movements with your opposite arm and leg. If you want, you can do this exercise next to a sturdy chair and place your free hand on its back for balance.

- **Wall push-ups**, which require that you stand in front of a wall at arm's length, place your palms flat upon it, making sure that they are shoulder-width apart, and bend your elbows slightly. Having done that, slowly bring your upper body close to the wall, keeping your feet together and unmoving. Then you push back out so that your arms straighten as if you were doing an actual push-up. Do 20 reps of this to work all the muscles running along your body.

- **Rock the boat**, where you stand with your back straight and your feet hip-width apart, then shift your body weight to your right leg and slightly raise your left leg off the ground. Hold this pose for a good 10 seconds before lowering your foot, shifting your weight the opposite way, and repeating everything. Keep going until you've done the same movement five times on each side.

The second skill you need to improve upon to get better at the choreographies you create for your dance cardio with rhythm sticks is memory. You have to be able to remember what moves you'll be doing as part of the choreography, after all. There are a couple of tricks you can use to improve your memory, luckily. Foremost among these is a method called chunking (Roberts, 2022). Chunking is a memorization method where you group a couple of different things, like moves that follow each other in a choreography sequence, and work on remembering them separately. Once you have different chunks down, you can string them together, which will make memorizing all the moves you have to do easier. If you're skeptical about how effective this would be, you should know that this is a skill you use every day. Say that you've got a new phone number and need to memorize it. Your new number is 917-844-7503. The easiest way to memorize this sequence of numbers is to do so in the chunks that they've been written down in, rather than as 9178447503 as a whole. Isn't that right?

As for how chunking works for cardio dance routines, you can divide your routines and choreographies into eight-count combos and focus on memorizing each combo first. You can then start stringing them together. At this stage, you can make use of the beat and rhythm of the song you're listening to, since the moves will match these elements of the music. You can also make up your own cues and counts. This can be as simple as coming up with new, personal names for your moves. It can also entail adding snaps where you need to and using any other sound cues, such as the clicking and clapping of your rhythm sticks. This is just one of the many reasons rhythm sticks are incredibly easy to incorporate into cardio dance choreographies.

However, this isn't the only type of workout where rhythm sticks can be an active and effective addition. There's also circuit training and more advanced training techniques such as high-intensity interval training (HIIT), as you will see in the coming chapters.

Chapter 8

Rhythm Sticks Circuit Training

Of all the different workout and training methods out there, circuit training is one of the most beneficial ones. It's so named because it involves rotating through a variety of different exercises that work the different parts of your body, thereby having you focus on changing muscle groups for short periods of time. The idea here is to complete the circuit multiple times, thus working all your muscles out properly and giving them enough time to rest in between, without taking passive rest—though you should absolutely take breaks between your sets. Sets are the sequences of fitness movements you do as part of your circuit training. Typically, you repeat these sets three to four times in your exercise session, making sure to take breaks in between. How long should your circuit-training sessions be, then? How should they work? Before we can start exploring the myriad of ways in which you can make rhythm sticks a part of your circuit training, we have to first understand how circuit training is supposed to work.

Introduction to Circuit Training

Circuit-training sessions make for ideal forms of exercise because they work the whole body, from top to bottom, without overtaxing any one part of the whole or any specific muscle groups. A typical session lasts somewhere between 30 and 45 minutes and keeps the rest periods between the sets relatively short. This is because the muscle groups you're not working while doing a specific move will be resting in between. So, if you have finished some arm exercises and are doing leg exercises now, you will be giving your arm muscles the time they need to rest. After that, you'll be able to circle back to your arm exercises.

Circuit training may sound quite familiar to you. However, there are different types of circuit training you could participate in if you wanted to. The chief circuit-training categories out there are (Gasnick, 2022):

- timed circuit

- repetition circuit

- sport-specific circuit

- competition circuit

In a timed circuit, you perform each circuit—meaning exercise moves making up your sets—in specific periods of time. Often, you are given between 30 and 90 seconds to complete, say, as many crunches as you can in a set, before being given the same amount of time to do as many lunges as you can. How much time you will be given for these sets—30, 60, or 90 seconds, or something in between—will depend on your fitness level, which your trainer and you will be able to discover beforehand using a fitness assessment, as you know.

In a repetition circuit, on the other hand, you will be focusing on repeating your chosen fitness movements a specific number of times. Usually, you'll be expected to do 10 to 15 repetitions of a movement, like squats for example. That done, you'll be able to move onto the next move in your sequences and do 10 to 15 reps of that one as well.

Timed circuit and repetition circuit are the most common versions of this kind of training. This is because sport-specific circuits and competition circuits are more targeted. Sport-specific circuits are designed to improve specific moves associated with a particular sport. If you were a basketball player, for example, your sport-specific circuit training might involve moves designed to improve your ability to jump, shoot a basket, and pass the ball. Meanwhile, competition circuits try to get you to complete as many repetitions of the moves you're given in a specific amount of time, say 30 seconds. As such, it's like an amalgamation of repetition and timed circuits.

Circuit training is incredibly popular and is an especially good option to pair with rhythm sticks. This is partly thanks to the fact that it gives you a full-body workout, which is what you want with rhythm sticks. It's also partly thanks to the unique benefits it has to offer people. You see, the series of movements that make up circuit-training sessions end up being derivatives of both cardiovascular and strength-training exercises. As such, they allow you to reap the benefits of both training models and help you to significantly increase your bodily strength. At the same time, they help you to lose weight, a known side effect of both exercise models. Of course, circuit training strengthens your heart and cardiovascular system too.

So, how do you combine circuit training with rhythm sticks? This depends on what type of circuit training you're opting for. As a general rule, repetition circuits and timed circuits work better with rhythm sticks than other types, with the former being the most preferred. Once you've chosen what kind of circuit training you want to do, you can choose which kinds of movements you want to make part of your sets and incorporate rhythm sticks into them.

Designing a Rhythm Sticks Circuit Training Workout

Let's say that you want to design your very own rhythm sticks circuit-training workout and that you've opted for the repetition type. What now? First, you have to choose which movements you'll be performing. Then, you'll have to decide how to do them with rhythm sticks. Finally, you'll want to decide how many reps and sets you want to do. One example of a very basic rhythm sticks circuit-training workout that'll last you a good 15 to 20 minutes and will be perfect for beginners might be (Anytime Fitness, 2022):

- Start your session with some warm-ups and stretches.

- Do step-ups with alternating feet for 60 seconds, raising your rhythm sticks into the air with each step and clapping them in front of you every time you step down.

- Rest for 30 seconds.

- Stand in a slight squat, hold your rhythm sticks in the middle, parallel to the ground, and start doing slow punches, picking up speed as you go, for 60 seconds straight. Make sure to keep to the rhythm of the song that's playing.

- Rest for 30 seconds.

- Do squats for 60 seconds straight, holding your rhythm sticks in front of your chest and clapping them both when you squat down and when you rise back up.

- Rest for 30 seconds.

- Do jumping jacks while doing overhead rhythm stick claps for 60 seconds straight.

- Rest for 30 seconds.

- Do full-body sit-ups, making sure to clap your rhythm sticks together once you get into a sitting position and to extend your arms back over your head when you lie back down, for 60 seconds straight.

- Rest for 30 seconds.

- Put your rhythm sticks to the side and start doing push-ups (or modified push-ups if the former are too difficult for you). Try to match your push-ups to the beat of the music you are listening to.

- Rest for 30 seconds.

- Again, leave your rhythm sticks on the ground next to you and lie on your back to do glute bridges. You can do this by lying face up with your knees bent and hip-width apart, keeping your feet firmly planted on the ground, then placing your hands on your stomach or your sides, or on the ground for greater balance. After that, lift your hips off the ground and squeeze your glutes as you go, pause for a beat, and lower your hips back down. You can keep going like this for 60 seconds straight.

- Rest for 30 seconds.

- Pick up your rhythm sticks again and do lunges for 60 seconds straight, clapping your sticks in front of you with each lunge.

- Rest for 30 seconds.

- Let go of your rhythm sticks and do a plank or modified plank. You can do the former by getting down on the floor so that you're on your forearms and toes, with your elbows directly beneath your shoulders. Keep your head relaxed, and have your forearms face forward and your eyes fixed on the floor. Tighten your abs and keep your back straight, your shoulders down, and your heels over the balls of your feet. You can do a modified plank by assuming the same position, but this time placing your knees on the ground as well, so that your weight is a little more distributed. In this case, make sure something soft like a yoga mat is beneath your legs. Whichever version of the plank you do, keep your pose for at least 30 seconds and try to go for 60 seconds if you can.

- Rest for 30 seconds.

- Pick up your rhythm sticks and do jumping jacks with overhead claps one last time for 30 seconds.

- End your session with some cool-downs and stretches.

Circuit Training for Total-Body Conditioning

This is of course just a very simple, beginner-level example of the kind of rhythm sticks circuit-training session you can craft for yourself. You can create longer and more complicated circuit-training routines. In the process, you'll be able to really improve your body's conditioning. The kind of circuit-training routine that will enable you to do this will, of course, last longer than 15–20 minutes. An example of such a routine that you can use to craft your very own might look like this (Anytime Fitness, 2023):

- Do a warm-up and stretching session.

- Do dumbbell rolls but use rhythm sticks instead. To do this you will need a bench of some sort that you can place your left knee and shin on, with your foot hanging off one end. Your left palm should also be placed on the bench, in front of and near to your knee. Your knee itself should be beneath your hips, just as your hand should be beneath your shoulder. If you've gotten that positioning right, then you can pick up your rhythm sticks in one hand. Investing in some weighted rhythm sticks might be a good idea for this particular exercise. Once you've picked your sticks up, you can extend the hand that's holding them to the ground, keep your back straight, and plant your right foot on the ground so that you remain balanced. Then, you can row your rhythm sticks toward your chest without rotating your body. What you want to do is drive your elbow toward the ceiling as you roll your sticks. You also want to pinch your shoulders. If you were holding dumbbells, you could get away with doing just 10 reps of this. Since you're holding rhythm sticks, you'll need to do 20, assuming you don't have weighted ones. Once your reps are done, you can switch positions and do the same move with your right arm, again going for 20 reps.

- Take a 30-second break.

- Do 20 reps of seated, single-arm overhead presses. To do this, you'll need to sit down on the ground, keeping your back straight, and extend your legs out at a 45-degree angle. Then, you'll grab your rhythm sticks in one hand and raise them so that they're level with your shoulders in a racked position. When you're ready, start pressing the rhythm sticks over your head while keeping your back straight. Lower them back down to their original position and keep going with the same movement.

- Take a 30-second break.

- Do step-ups for 30 seconds straight, clapping your rhythm sticks before your chest each time you step up and step down.

- Take a 30-second break.

- Do 15 reps per foot of anti-rotation presses, which you can do by getting down into a half-kneeling position while grabbing your rhythm sticks by both hands, so that they are parallel to the ground. Keep the sticks close to your chest as you rise up. As you sink back down, push the sticks away from your chest and tighten your arm muscles as you do so. Keep going like that until your reps are done.

- Take a 30-second break.

- Put your rhythm sticks to the side and do push-ups or modified push-ups for 60 seconds straight.

- Take a 30-second break.

- Do burpees for 30 seconds. You will need to let go of your rhythm sticks for this exercise too. Place your hands on the ground after getting into a squat position. Then step back into a plank position. Hold the pose for a beat, then step back to your original crouch position. Then get to your feet, before dropping back down to your original pose and repeating the moves.

- Do jumping jacks with rhythm sticks for 60 seconds straight.

- Take a 30-second break.

- Do squats for 60 seconds straight.

- Do sit-ups with rhythm sticks for 60 seconds straight.

- Take a 30-second break.

- Repeat this entire sequence twice more.

- Do your cool-down and stretching exercises and call it a day.

Chapter 9

Advanced Rhythm Sticks

Cardio Techniques

Rhythm sticks can also be incorporated into more intense, advanced workout routines and styles. In the process, they can become a part of your journey to really push your limits, improve your strength, agility, and conditioning, and keep yourself in peak physical condition. For this, though, you will need to learn some advanced rhythm sticks cardio and strength-training moves. The primary moves you will thus end up adding to your repertoire are:

- **Windshield wipers**, where you hold either a quarter of a squat or full squat position before a rhythm sticks drum—meaning a Pilates ball in a bucket—to do side crunches around it, tapping the sides of said drum as though your sticks were windshield wipers.

- **Squat and hit**, which will require you to squat down and hit either the ground or your drum.

- **Click jacks**, which are those jumping jacks that require doing clicks or claps with your rhythm sticks while you jump.

- **Lunges and click squats**, which is a move where you do lunges while performing clicks in front, overhead, and to your sides in sequence with each lunge.

- **Grapevine**, which is a move where you jump left to hit your neighbor's drum for four beats, then jump back to your own drum to strike another four beats there.

- **Crossovers**, where you will click right, left, right, and then left on your own drum in rapid succession.

- **Circle pattern around the world**, where you either hop or walk around your drum, landing single or double hits on it as you go, until you've come full circle.

You can incorporate such moves into your workout sessions to make things even more intense. You can also go for something like HIIT to really get your blood pumping and get some results.

High Intensity Interval Training With Rhythm Sticks

First things first, what exactly is HIIT? HIIT, or high-intensity interval training as it is otherwise known, is a type of interval training. What does that mean? Interval training sessions are workout sessions that involve short bursts of really intense activity. This activity gets your heart rate to climb incredibly quickly, which is why it's done in bursts. Naturally, it comes with an array of benefits all its own. For example, HIIT is known to help people build strength. It can boost and support your metabolism in some surprising ways too. This is to be expected given how the workout increases your stamina. As for the reason it's able to do this, this is thanks to HIIT pushing your body into what's known as the anaerobic zone. The anaerobic zone happens when your heart starts performing at 80–90% capacity (Circle Health Group, n.d.). In other words, it's when your heart is beating faster than it normally—or even ever—does. Obviously, such speeds aren't sustainable in the long term, but in the short term, they're quite doable. Not only that, but they can be quite beneficial for your cardiovascular system too, as they will strengthen it and increase its stamina as well.

One of the foremost advantages of HIIT is that it can burn 13 calories per minute. That's a lot of calories and a lot of fat, when you think about it, which is why this type of workout can be great for weight loss and managing conditions such as obesity. Another reason for this is that, like strength training, HIIT workouts make your body keep burning fat long after your workout sessions are over. One of the most surprising benefits of the workout, though, is that it keeps you young on a very physical and literal level. There's a hormone called the human growth hormone (HGH). HIIT stimulates this hormone, making your body release a ton of it while you're working out. Since HGH is primarily a hormone that your body releases when you're in your adolescence, this results in an interesting side effect: It makes you look—and feel—a lot younger than you are. Coupled with the health-raising effects, then, HIIT workouts can make for some pretty surprising changes in your life.

So, how exactly does a HIIT workout go? That depends entirely on what kinds of exercise moves you want to make use of, but a very basic, 19-minute-long version of the routine might look like this:

- Do your warm-up and stretching exercises.

- Do two sets of high knees, each of which will take you 20 seconds, while either tapping your knees against your rhythm sticks each time you raise them, or rapidly clapping the sticks before you as you go.

- Do two sets of plank punches, where you alternately raise one hand off the ground while maintaining the plank position to punch forward.

- Do two sets of jumping jacks with clicks.

- Do two sets of lateral shuffles, where you rapidly clap your rhythm sticks as you go.

- Rest for 60 seconds.

- Keeping your feet together, jump from left to right without stopping for 60 seconds straight, while doing side claps with your rhythm sticks with each landing.

- Do two sets of sit-ups, making sure to clap your rhythm sticks once you are sitting up and extend your arms fully over your head when you lay back down.

- Drop your rhythm sticks and do two sets of push-ups or modified push-ups, where you rest your knees on the ground to distribute your weight a little more.

- Do two sets of jumping jacks with overhead claps.

- Take a 60-second break.

- Do two sets of burpees without stopping.

- Do two sets of squats, doing side and front claps every time you drop into a squat.

- Do two sets of lunges, doing side and front claps every time you drop into a lunge.

- Do two sets of Russian twists, where you sit on the floor and bring your legs up to the tabletop position, lean back so that your body forms a sort of V-like shape, tighten your core muscles, and start twisting from side to side. Keep your legs immobile as you do this and perform side claps with your rhythm sticks each time you twist to the side.

- Take a break for 60 seconds.

- Do two sets of mountain climbers, which is a move where you drop your rhythm sticks temporarily and put both your hands and feet on the ground, with your right foot next to your right hand and your left foot extended before you. Then you leap to bring your right foot back level with where your left foot was, while moving your left foot next to your left hand. Keep going like that without pausing in between the motions.

- Stand with one foot before you and the other behind you and start jumping. With each jump, switch the positions of your feet. Do one clap when you're airborne and one clap when you land. Keep going like that, as fast as you can, for 60 seconds straight.

- Do two steps of box jumps, which you will need a step or box to perform. Get behind a sturdy box and jump onto it. Clap your rhythm sticks the moment you land, then jump back down and clap your sticks once more. Keep going like that, without pausing between your moves, for 60 seconds straight.

- Stop and do your cool-down and stretching exercises.

Pushing Limits and Breaking Plateaus

HIIT and other similar advanced and intense workout techniques are your best bet for pushing and breaking your limits and plateaus. They essentially enable you to discover what your limits are and have you go past them bit by bit, since they involve spurts of heavy effort. The key word there is "spurts." Doing short bursts of intense activity, you see, makes the pain and exhaustion that come with it a great deal more bearable.

The short duration for which you have to push yourself makes you more amenable to doing so. "It's just for 5 more minutes" creates a whole different psychological effect than, say, "I have to keep doing this for another 40 minutes," as anyone would agree.

The duration of your workouts then, and the intensity at which you go at them, are intimately connected. The way you view those intervals of time can help you to keep pushing yourself and discovering things about yourself that you maybe didn't know. There are other techniques you can use to accomplish this, though. One is setting goals for yourself, which can be immeasurably effective in motivating you, as you'll see in the coming chapters. Another is finding an uplifting, motivating, or encouraging mantra for yourself. Finding a mantra will help you during intense workout sessions for two reasons. The first is that it will keep you in a more positive mindset, allowing you to keep your motivation levels high. The second is that it will distract you from the pain, for lack of a better word, that accompanies your workout sessions. At the very least, it'll direct your attention away from your burning muscles and how hard your heart is beating at that moment, thereby making it possible for you to keep going for just a little bit longer.

Another thing that can achieve this same result is taking care to express gratitude for the workout that you are physically able to do, even and especially if you have any physical limitations that you have to factor in. Being able to workout is a great blessing because it means you're able to keep moving as you want. You're able to strengthen your body and support it as it serves you.

The intense exercise session you're putting yourself through is a mark of how strong, healthy, and capable your body is; hence, any pain you're feeling in that moment is as well.

Chapter 10:

Cooling Down and Stretching

You already know that properly warming up is incredibly important. You might be thinking that cool-downs aren't quite that vital. If that's the case, then I'm sorry to tell you that you are wrong. Cool-downs are a vital part of any workout session, as are post-workout stretches. This is because these two things give your heart and body the post-workout recovery time they need, before making them go back to their everyday work and activities. This not only prevents wear and tear, but also makes it possible for you to have a more enjoyable rest of your day, rather than an out-of-breath and crampy one.

The Importance of Cooling Down

All of this may sound just a little too generic to you at the moment though, and you might be confused as to why, exactly, cool-downs are as important as warm-ups. If that's the case, let's quickly take a look at the many reasons you want to take those 10 to 15 minutes after you're finished with your official workout to do cool-down and stretching exercises.

The first reason cool-downs are important is that they help alleviate the stress that workouts put on your body (Carter, 2022). Physically speaking, working out is a stressful thing for the human body. It pushes the body, tests its limits, and at times makes it go beyond them. Speaking on solely a musculoskeletal level, your muscles basically tear during your workout session. Afterward they repair themselves and become even stronger than before. That's why working out makes you stronger. When you cool down after your workouts, you actually make it easier for your muscles to do this. You give them the rest, space, and time they need to recuperate and start knitting themselves back together.

At the same time, you end up improving your circulation by doing cool-down exercises. As a result, your body is able to expel more wasteful by-products from your body than it ordinarily would be able to. With the removal of these by-products, your muscles and joints start feeling better. They have an easier time building themselves back up and feel a lot less stiff than before.

Increasing your flexibility is also important for eliminating this stiffness from your body. The best way you can do this is by following your cool-downs with some stretching exercises, because those impact your overall flexibility, as you know. That being the case, let's take a closer look at what kinds of cool-down moves you can turn to.

Relaxation and Stretching Exercises With Rhythm Sticks

Some of the best, most relaxing cool-down and stretching exercises you can do with rhythm sticks are (Jackson-Gibson, 2020):

- **Child's pose**, where you get on all fours, sit your butt on your heels, and stretch your hands forward, trying to reach as far ahead as possible with your rhythm sticks in your hands. You need to drop your head down in between your shoulders as you do this and try to really feel the stretch in your upper body and arms. Hold the pose for between 60 and 90 seconds for the best effect.

- **Pigeon pose**, where you get on all fours again and place your right knee forward, trying to rotate your external hip as much as possible while laying your leg down on the ground and lowering your chest so that the stretch goes all the way down to your butt. Your hands should be clasped together on the ground with your rhythm sticks held in between them, perpendicular to the ground. They should be just in front of your head and should not be touching your face.

- **Behind the back grip stretch**, where you sit down on the ground and press your shoulders down and squeeze your shoulder blades together. Holding a rhythm stick in one hand, you should bend your elbows behind your back and try to extend the rhythm stick past the elbow of the opposite arm.

- **Sumo squat stretch**, where you stand with your feet hip-width apart, drop into a squat, and let your hands, which will be holding your rhythm sticks, dangle down between your feet. Then you'll bring your elbows above your knees and press your knees outward, clapping your rhythm sticks all the while.

- **Overhead shoulder stretch**, where you'll raise your arms above your head, with a rhythm stick in your left hand. Next, bend that arm behind your back, grab your rhythm stick from the other end with your right hand, and pull to extend and stretch the arm. Hold that pose for 30 seconds, before switching hands and repeating the move on the opposite side.

- **Standing one-legged ankle twist**, where you stand with your feet close together, raise a knee to your chest, and draw figure-eights with your foot, counting to four by clapping your rhythm sticks in front of you as you go, then switching feet and repeating the same move.

Chapter 11:

Incorporating Rhythm Sticks Cardio Into Your Daily Life

It's a well-established fact by now that working out is a very necessary part of your life—or that it should be, anyway. Working out can be hard to do though, especially if you're not the biggest fan of physical activity in general. Typically, there are two reasons, that is to say excuses, why seniors avoid working out: that they do not have the time for it, and that they find it hard to remain motivated enough to keep going. Luckily, there are some easy-to-implement solutions you can use to address both these issues. What exactly are these solutions and how can you make use of them? Let's find out!

Integrating Exercise Into Your Daily Routine

It's true that you might be leading a very hectic lifestyle and that finding the time to work out might be rather difficult for you. Difficult doesn't mean impossible, though. It just means you are going to have to be a little more creative and thoughtful in organizing your day-to-day schedule so that you can make the time you need for exercise. One way you can do this is to actually schedule your workouts in your calendar. A lot of the time, it's not your busy schedule that's to blame for your being unable to work out (*9 Ways to Make Time*, 2022); it's poor planning. Trying to squeeze too many things into one day or going about your day without planning a schedule can result in your activities taking much longer than anticipated. This can, in turn, result in you having to push back certain things, including that workout session you wanted to do. If you schedule your workout in advance, though, and plan out the rest of your week, you can avoid this problem. As a result, you'll be able to get much better at time management too and probably end up with a lot more free time than you used to have, which you'll be able to use however you'd like.

Another thing that might help you is to schedule 10- or 15-minute-long workout sessions during the day, as opposed to 30-minute ones. It doesn't matter how long you work out for in a single go, so long as you meet your 150 minutes per week requirement. You can squeeze in 5-minute-long sessions throughout your day if you want, and that would be perfectly fine. Let's face it, no matter how busy a life you lead, you can always find 5 minutes to spare. This is especially true when you're waiting for the laundry to be done or for your food to finish cooking.

One thing that can help you even more is to start waking earlier than you used to. This doesn't mean you should forgo some of your sleep, of course. You should still get all the sleep that your body needs. It does, however, mean that you can create some dramatic changes in your day-to-day schedule by waking up just 30 minutes earlier and working out for 15 minutes in the morning. You'd be surprised how much free time such a small act can potentially give you.

Joining a group class or activity can further help you find time to work out, or at least be motivated enough to do so. Group activities tend to be a lot more fun than solo workout sessions. So, going to a gym or community center and finding a rhythm stick group session may end up providing you with a very entertaining and social way to spend your time. That your workout sessions will be entertaining activities you can do with friends or become environments where you can make new friends will make you like and want to go to them even more. Thus, the "I don't have time for it" excuse will start losing some of its power. Before you know it, you'll be looking forward to your group classes and going to them as regularly as possible.

Staying Motivated

Another important reason older adults often don't work out is that they find it hard to motivate themselves to do so. Again, though, this is the kind of problem that's relatively easy to solve, at least when you know how to approach it. One easy way to motivate yourself might be to give yourself an actual reward that you would genuinely enjoy. Let's say that you are really into a TV show, to the point that you constantly want to binge it. If that's the case, you can make watching an episode of that show into a reward you treat yourself to after your workout sessions. This will cause an inextricable link to form between the two activities. Once that happens, you'll start looking forward to your workouts, if only so you can get your reward. After a while, your body will get used to the surge of endorphins that come with working out and start craving the good feelings they bring with them. This will only increase your motivation to keep going. Pretty soon you won't even need your reward, but you can certainly keep receiving it, if only as an added bonus.

Another very motivating thing you can do is to visualize the many benefits that rhythm sticks cardio and working out in general have to offer you. You've uncovered a great number of these benefits throughout the course of this book. So, why not visualize yourself living those benefits? Picturing yourself leading a more active lifestyle, where you have greater freedom and mobility because you have a stronger and healthier body, can be incredibly motivating. It can remind you precisely why you are exercising and drive you to keep going, even when the going gets tough. It can enable you to push past your boundaries and limits, leading you to discover hidden strengths and sides that you didn't know you had.

A final thing you can do to increase your motivation and make sure it lasts is to find your very own fitness group or tribe, so to speak. Working out with other people is always more fun than working out alone. Beyond that, working out with others can motivate you to keep going and do your absolute best. This is a bit like how you get more into the working spirit when you go into the office and see everyone else hard at work too. Their focus and enthusiasm for the job proves catching in this case, making you work hard too. In group sessions, though, this effect is even more accentuated because of the people you are surrounded by. This form of external motivation can be just the burst of encouragement you need. It can both ensure that you keep going to class after class and session after session, and that you keep testing your limits in class. Add to that the friendships that you can forge in class, and it's easy to see how the very act of going to group rhythm sticks sessions and classes can be hugely motivating.

Maintaining a Lifelong Fitness Journey

Rhythm sticks cardio isn't one of those activities that you try once and then quickly forget about. Instead, it's the sort of thing that quickly gets its hooks into you. It proves as entertaining as it is beneficial, as good for your mental health as it is for your physical health. Once you experience these effects for yourself, quitting the sport becomes rather hard, if not downright impossible to do.

This is what makes rhythm sticks cardio a very easy workout routine to turn into a lifelong fitness journey. It's the kind of sport that sticks with you no matter what age you are. It's the kind of thing that you can enjoy as part of your regular life, without having to learn any skills or techniques that are overly complicated, or get equipment that is bulky and expensive. Instead, rhythm sticks cardio is one of the easiest sports in the world, not to mention one of the most varied, as you have already seen.

There are many ways in which you can incorporate rhythm sticks into your life, and the one you go with depends entirely on what your preferences, tastes, and desires are. Put simply, rhythm sticks cardio is the kind of workout that has something to offer to anybody and everybody. It's especially well suited to older adults given how easy to do and low impact it is. Hence, it is the kind of workout that you can embrace wholeheartedly and enjoy for many healthy, strong years to come.

Conclusion

There are many different sports and workout routines for you to choose from, as you know, and it's important for both your physical and mental health that you do choose one. This makes an abundance of sense considering the benefits that working out has to offer you. From keeping your body strong and mobile to boosting your immune system and increasing your flexibility, the simple act of staying active is the key to living a long and fulfilling life. That being said, there are clearly some forms of exercise that are better for older adults than others. Low-impact forms of exercise that are as easy to pick up as they can be challenging are foremost among such exercise routines. There are a number of such exercises, of course, but after all that you've learned and discovered, it's clear to see that rhythm sticks cardio is among the best of them, if not the best.

If you've made it to this part of *Rhythm Sticks Cardio for Seniors,* you are well aware of this fact by now. You're also aware of just how much fun you can have by getting into this sport. The one question you may have, then, is where you might do so. Luckily, this is an easy enough question to answer: You can likely find rhythm sticks cardio in a nearby gym, senior center, or even community center. All you have to do is pay them a visit or look at their website, if you are tech savvy, to check and find classes that work with your schedule. In the meantime, you can always start practicing at home to at least learn some of the basic moves. That way, you can quickly get into the rhythm of things when you go in for group sessions and really start enjoying yourself.

Of course, you'll end up learning and discovering a great many more things about this unique sport once you have gotten into it. But that's only to be expected in an exercise model as unique and creative as rhythm sticks cardio. Let's face it, though, that'll only be part of the fun, once you've chosen your sticks, put on your workout gear, and headed out. So, what are you waiting for?

References

Admin. *Aerobic exercises for seniors: Everything you should know.* (2020, March 25). Athulya. https://www.athulyaliving.com/blogs/aerobic-exercises-for-seniors-everything-you-should-know.php

Alricsson, M., & Werner, S. (2004). The effect of pre-season dance training on physical indices and back pain in elite cross-country skiers: A prospective controlled intervention study. *British Journal of Sports Medicine, 38*(2), 148–153. https://doi.org/10.1136/bjsm.2002.2402

Alzheimer's Association. (n.d.). Can *Alzheimer's disease be prevented?* https://www.alz.org/alzheimers-dementia/research_progress/prevention

Anytime Fitness. (2022, December 2). *15-minute beginner circuit workout.* https://www.anytimefitness.com/ccc/15-minute-circuit-workout-perfect-for-beginners

Anytime Fitness. (2023, February 2). *30-minute full body circuit workout.* https://www.anytimefitness.com/ccc/workouts/30-minute-full-body-circuit-workout/

Baarøy, F.-A. (2020, August 30). A *sense of rhythm – why do we have it and what does it mean to us?* RITMO

Centre for Interdisciplinary Studies in Rhythm, Time and Motion, University of Oslo. https://www.uio.no/ritmo/english/news-and-events/news/2018/a-sense-of-rhythm---why-do-we-have-it-and-what-doe.html#:~:text=%E2%80%9CMany%20people%20probably%20don

Barr, C. (2023, June 22). *Cardio drumming: A fun and energizing workout for 2023*. Sonic Function. https://sonicfunction.com/cardio-drumming/

Beavers, K. M., Ambrosius, W. T., Rejeski, W. J., Burdette, J. H., Walkup, M. P., Sheedy, J. L., Nesbit, B. A., Gaukstern, J. E., Nicklas, B. J., & Marsh, A. P. (2017). Effect of exercise type during intentional weight loss on body composition in older adults with obesity. *Obesity, 25*(11), 1823–1829. https://doi.org/10.1002/oby.21977

Bedosky, L. (2022, April 22). *The best core exercises for seniors*. Get Healthy U | Chris Freytag. https://gethealthyu.com/best-core-exercises-for-seniors/

Bennington-Castro, J. (2022, September 6). *Detecting and diagnosing depression: It can look different in men and women and in teenagers, too*. Everyday Health. https://www.everydayhealth.com/depression/guide/symptoms/

Carter, S. (2022, October 22). *Why it's important to cool down after exercise, according to the science*. Live Science. https://www.livescience.com/why-its-

important-to-cool-down-after-exercise-
according-to-the-science

Centers for Disease Control and Prevention. (2021,
February 17). *How much physical activity do older
adults need?*
https://www.cdc.gov/physicalactivity/basics/o
lder_adults/index.htm

Centers for Disease Control and Prevention. (2023,
March 24). *Keep on your feet—preventing older adult
falls.*
https://www.cdc.gov/injury/features/older-
adult-falls/index.html

Circle Health Group. (n.d.). *10 benefits of high-intensity
interval training (HIIT).*
https://www.circlehealthgroup.co.uk/health-
matters/womens-health/10-benefits-of-hiit

Cleveland Clinic. (2019, August 1). *How can you avoid
muscle loss as you age?*
https://health.clevelandclinic.org/how-can-
you-avoid-muscle-loss-as-you-age/

Condran, C. (2019, November 20). *Rhythm sticks routine
– Uptown Funk #physed* [Video]. YouTube.
https://www.youtube.com/watch?v=wbZmFP
NLJ2g&ab_channel=ChanceCondran

Conghalaigh, J. (2019, September 15). *This is your brain
on drumming.* Medium.
https://medium.com/swlh/this-is-your-brain-
on-drumming-8ed6eaf314c4

Cordier, A. (2018, February 9). *5 reasons why warm up exercises are important.* Fit Athletic Club. https://fitathletic.com/5-reasons-warm-exercises-important/

Easy Leg Exercises for Seniors to Improve Mobility and Balance. (2021, March 27). Holiday Retirement. https://www.holidayretirement.com/easy-leg-exercises-for-seniors-to-improve-mobility/

Fahmy, R. (n.d.). *Exercise programming for seniors.* National Academy of Sports Medicine. https://blog.nasm.org/exercise-programming-for-older-adults

Falk, M. (2022, May 17). *The best cardio exercises to mix into your at-home workouts.* Shape. https://www.shape.com/fitness/cardio/best-cardio-exercises-at-home

Fatima, S. (2023, March 3). *Coordination exercises for older adults.* Sugarfit. https://www.sugarfit.com/blog/coordination-exercises-for-older-adults/

Fetters, K. A. (2018, April 27). *Cardio for seniors: Best advice.* SilverSneakers. https://www.silversneakers.com/blog/the-best-cardio-advice-youre-not-taking/

Fitness for seniors: Tailor exercise to individuals. (2013, April 8). *The Denver Post.* https://www.denverpost.com/2013/04/08/fitness-for-seniors-tailor-exercise-to-individuals/

Freytag, C. (2022, February 4). *20-minute strength training workout for seniors.* Verywell Fit. https://www.verywellfit.com/20-minute-senior-weight-training-workout-3498676

Gasnick, K. (2022, May 31). *Circuit training: Everything you need to know.* Verywell Health. https://www.verywellhealth.com/what-is-circuit-training-5224393

Gomez-Pinilla, F., & Hillman, C. (2013). The influence of exercise on cognitive abilities. *Comprehensive Physiology, 3*(1). https://doi.org/10.1002/cphy.c110063

Hanna, K. A. (2022, October 2). *How to make rhythm sticks.* FeltMagnet. https://feltmagnet.com/crafts/How-to-Make-Rhythm-Sticks

Horvath-Krol, D. (2020, September 20). *How to booty pop.* WikiHow. https://www.wikihow.com/Booty-Pop

How to do a jumping jack. (2019). *The New York Times.* https://www.nytimes.com/guides/well/activity/how-to-do-a-jumping-jack

Iliades, C. (2018, January 30). *8 ways strength training boosts your health and fitness.* Everyday Health. https://www.everydayhealth.com/fitness/add-strength-training-to-your-workout.aspx

Jackson-Gibson, A. (2020, July 30). *14 best cool down exercises to recover and stretch after a workout.*

Prevention.
https://www.prevention.com/fitness/g334336
18/cool-down-exercises/

Leslie. (2014, August 25). *Let's play with rhythm sticks!* Musical Bridges Music Therapy. https://www.musicalbridgesmt.com/2014/08/25/lets-play-with-rhythm-sticks/

Loncaric, D. (2022, February 22). *What is cardio drumming?* DRUM! Magazine. https://drummagazine.com/cardio-drumming/

Loudin, A. (2023, March 15). *A 19-minute HIIT workout for beginners.* The New York Times. https://www.nytimes.com/2023/03/15/well/move/hiit-workout-beginner.html

Manor, B. (2019, October 22). *Preventing falls in older adults: Multiple strategies are better.* Harvard Health Publishing. https://www.health.harvard.edu/blog/preventing-falls-in-older-adults-multiple-strategies-are-better-2019102218085

Martinez, M. (2017, April 13). *Rhythm stick routine- we will rock you* [Video]. YouTube. https://www.youtube.com/watch?v=yefws73QN1A&ab_channel=MaresaMartinez

May, K. (2019, December 27). *5 ways seniors can stay safe while exercising.* Home Care Assistance. https://www.homecareassistanceamarillo.com/how-can-seniors-stay-safe-when-exercising/

Mayo Clinic Staff. (2021, October 6). *Aerobic exercise: How to warm up and cool down*. Mayo Clinic. https://www.mayoclinic.org/healthy-lifestyle/fitness/in-depth/exercise/art-20045517#

Mayo Clinic Staff. (2022, February 23). *Slide show: A guide to basic stretches*. Mayo Clinic. https://www.mayoclinic.org/healthy-lifestyle/fitness/multimedia/stretching/sls-20076840?s=6

Mcleod, J. C., Stokes, T., & Phillips, S. M. (2019). Resistance exercise training as a primary countermeasure to age-related chronic disease. *Frontiers in Physiology*, *10*. https://doi.org/10.3389/fphys.2019.00645

Merom, D., Grunseit, A., Eramudugolla, R., Jefferis, B., Mcneill, J., & Anstey, K. J. (2016). Cognitive benefits of social dancing and walking in old age: The Dancing Mind randomized controlled trial. *Frontiers in Aging Neuroscience*, *8*. https://www.frontiersin.org/articles/10.3389/fnagi.2016.00026/full

Momma, H., Kawakami, R., Honda, T., & Sawada, S. S. (2022). Muscle-strengthening activities are associated with lower risk and mortality in major non-communicable diseases: a systematic review and meta-analysis of cohort studies. *British Journal of Sports Medicine*, *56*(13), 755–763. https://doi.org/10.1136/bjsports-2021-105061

Montecino-Rodriguez, E., Berent-Maoz, B., & Dorshkind, K. (2013). Causes, consequences, and reversal of immune system aging. *Journal of Clinical Investigation*, *123*(3), 958–965. https://doi.org/10.1172/jci64096

National Health Service. (2021, August 4). *Physical activity guidelines for adults aged 19 to 64*. https://www.nhs.uk/live-well/exercise/exercise-guidelines/physical-activity-guidelines-for-adults-aged-19-to-64/

9 ways to make time for exercise with a busy schedule. (2022, September 8). Polar. https://www.polar.com/blog/9-ways-how-to-make-time-for-exercise/

Ollie. (2021, April 27). *Squats for elderly people 2022*. Wise Fitness Academy. https://wisefitnessacademy.com/squats-for-elderly/

Prvulovic, T. (2023, February 6). *Exercise recovery time over 50*. Second Wind Movement. https://secondwindmovement.com/exercise-recovery-time/

Ramos, N. (2020, November 7). *Rhythm sticks routine (PE III)- Dance again by Jennifer Lopez* [Video]. YouTube. https://www.youtube.com/watch?v=lOzv5dhy77E&ab_channel=NoemiRamos

Ramos-Campo, D. J., Andreu Caravaca, L., Martínez-Rodríguez, A., & Rubio-Arias, J. Á. (2021).

Effects of resistance circuit-based training on body composition, strength and cardiorespiratory fitness: A systematic review and meta-analysis. *Biology*, *10*(5), 377. https://doi.org/10.3390/biology10050377

Revelation Wellness. (2022, March 23). *40-min drumsticks cardio workout w/ Amia Freeman* [Video]. YouTube. https://www.youtube.com/watch?v=m31O5O 9KhPc&ab_channel=RevelationWellness

Richardson, G. (2020, January 28). *Cardio drumming – Exercise and improve your stamina in the process.* Zing Instruments. https://zinginstruments.com/cardio-drumming/

Roberts, C. (2022, December 16). *5 tips to help you remember choreography.* STEEZY. https://www.steezy.co/posts/how-to-memorize-choreography

Runner Bean Health & Fitness. (2021, August 2). *STIX | 4 minute sticks workout | Full body cardio sticks workout* [Video]. YouTube. https://www.youtube.com/watch?v=GgLY39 HSpA8&ab_channel=RunnerBeanHealth%26Fi tness

Seegert, L. (2021, June 1). *4 ways exercise helps fight aging.* Time. https://time.com/6053055/how-exercise-fights-aging/

Shawley, J. (2020, January 13). *Learning moves & patterns for fitness drumming in PE.* Gopher. https://blog.gophersport.com/learning-moves-patterns-for-fitness-drumming-in-pe/

Spotebi. (2015, December 31). *Side shuffle | Illustrated exercise guide.* https://www.spotebi.com/exercise-guide/side-shuffle/

Suzuki, W. (2017). *The brain-changing benefits of exercise* [Video]. TED. https://www.ted.com/talks/wendy_suzuki_the_brain_changing_benefits_of_exercise

Tucker, L. A. (2017). Physical activity and telomere length in U.S. men and women: An NHANES investigation. *Preventive Medicine, 100,* 145–151. https://doi.org/10.1016/j.ypmed.2017.04.027

Volpi, E., Nazemi, R., & Fujita, S. (2004). Muscle tissue changes with aging. *Current Opinion in Clinical Nutrition and Metabolic Care, 7*(4), 405–410. https://doi.org/10.1097/01.mco.0000134362.76653.b2

Watson, S. (2014, July 21). *Balance training.* WebMD. https://www.webmd.com/fitness-exercise/a-z/balance-training

Why posture matters. (2017, January 4). Harvard Health. https://www.health.harvard.edu/staying-healthy/why-good-posture-matters

Working it out: Researchers find exercise may help fight depression in seniors. (2019, February 7). ScienceDaily. https://www.sciencedaily.com/releases/2019/02/190207111309.htm

Young, M. (2021a, June 23). *4 ways to do a squat.* SilverSneakers. https://www.silversneakers.com/blog/woyw-squat-older-adults-ways-do-it/

Young, M. (2021b, June 29). *Master the move: Reverse lunge.* SilverSneakers. https://www.silversneakers.com/blog/woyw-master-move-reverse-lunge/9

9 798822 310578